THE ENGLISH SPEAKER'S GUIDE TO

DOCTORS & HOSPITALS IN MEXICO

BY

MONICA RIX PAXSON

AND

LUIS FELIPE GARCIA PEREZ

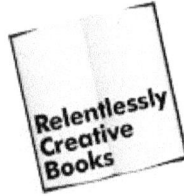

1st Edition

The English Speaker's Guide to Doctors & Hospitals in Mexico

by Monica Rix Paxson & Luis Felipe Garcia Perez

Copyright © 2014

ISBN 978-0-9895406-7-4

Book Website: http://medicaltourismsouth.com/
Monica Rix Paxson's Website: http://monicarixpaxson.com/
Published by Relentlessly Creative Books, USA
Publisher's Website: http://relentlesslycreative.com/
Publisher's Email: books@relentlesslycreative.com

Other titles by Monica Rix Paxson
The English Speaker's Guide to Medical Care in Mexico
The English Speaker's Guide to Social Networking & Expat Groups in Mexico
Talking2Trees & Other True Transdimensional Tales
The Tellstars in Orbit
The Fabulous Money-Making Garage Sale Kit
Dead Mars, Dying Earth
The Trouble with Level Three

Other titles by Luis Felipe Garcia Perez
Flippy's Life Lessons

Disclaimer

The English Speaker's Guide to Doctors & Hospitals in Mexico is not intended to give medical advice. It is a reference guide that is designed to help readers find resources that provide the care they are looking for. This book provides listings for informational purposes only. People who are using this resource are responsible for using their own judgment to determine the medical/surgical qualifications of any individual, medical service provider or medical care facility listed. Monica Rix Paxson nor Luis Felipe Garcia Perez have not independently reviewed or confirmed the information provided by the governmental, publishing or medical organizations who provided information for this publication and do not warrant the accuracy of the information provided in this directory. In no event shall Monica Rix Paxson, Luis Felipe Garcia Perez, Relentlessly Creative Books, their web publishers or distributors be liable for any decision made or taken by you based on this information. Because Monica Rix Paxson and Luis Felipe Garcia Perez are researchers and writers and not healthcare providers, they will not answer medical questions. Your questions about your health should be directed to the many medical professionals listed in this book.

TABLE OF CONTENTS

INTRODUCTION

Mexico has one of the most interesting, complex and unexpectedly enlightened medical systems in the world. From its long history of herbalism and healing that predates the Aztec empire, to using the most advanced technological and surgical techniques available today, the doctors and hospitals of Mexico save lives and make whole many of us who seek help because we are ill or injured.

Yet despite Mexico's 4000 plus private and public hospitals and countless medical doctors and dentists, there are still unique challenges for we foreigners. When the need for medical care arises, we are filled with questions: Where do I go to find the care that I need? Where can we find a doctor or dentist that understands English? Where is the nearest specialist? Where do we go in an emergency?

In my book *The English Speaker's Guide to Medical Care in Mexico*, my goal was to give expats and tourists an overview of how the medical system in Mexico works (and how it sometimes doesn't) rather than to make referrals to specific practitioners. However, with over a million English speakers living in Mexico and more arriving daily, the need for information isn't just theoretical. For example, if you are sick or in pain, you need help immediately. Information about where to go for the care you need is essential and sometimes urgent. This book is a go-to resource for immediate information.

The doctors and hospitals in this guide have been recommended by sources we trust. The vast majority of physicians listed speak English, although their proficiency varies. In some instances we have listed doctors and hospitals where only Spanish is spoken (as noted)

because they are in location with few other resources. The headings indicate areas of specialization, and when a physician has more than one specialty, we have attempted to list him or her under all the appropriate headings.

As my co-author, Luis Felipe Garcia Perez, and I found while researching the information for this directory, building a database of English-speaking practitioners, and hospitals that employ English speaking staff is not just a huge undertaking, it is like herding cats. No matter how hard we try, we cannot personally vet thousands of doctors and keep all of their contact information up-to-date, but we try our best.

Nor can we guarantee what your experience will be. For example, we cannot be certain that the one English-speaker on staff will be on duty when you arrive. There are limits to the magic we can perform. For example we cannot provide a list of specialists in a town when the sum total of available medical services may be one small hospital, a handful of general practitioners and a dentist. As in the USA and Canada, some areas of Mexico are very well served and others very poorly.

So, what follows represents new beginnings for all of us. For you it is an introduction to specific doctors, dentists and hospitals and we would hope initiate the beginning of new professional relationships. For us, it is the fulfillment of a long-held vision to bring together the various threads of Mexico's diverse and divergent medical community so that hopefully you can find what you need when and where you need it.

We welcome your contributions, updates and feedback.

Monica Rix Paxson
Author, *The English Speaker's Guide to Medical Care in Mexico*
Medical Facilitator for Mexperience.com
email: facilitator@medicaltourismhelpdesk.com

ACAPULCO

ANESTHESIOLOGISTS

Dra. María Luisa Elizabeth Anaya Ponce
(Anesthesiologist and Surgeon)
Torre Médica Cristóbal Colón
2da Calle de Cristóbal Colón 1623 int. 301
Fracc. Magallanes
Acapulco, Guerrero
Tel.: (744) 485-4109
Cel.: (744) 449-2758

CARDIOLOGISTS

Dr. Norberto Matadamas
Internal Medicine, Cardiology
Address: Calle Wilfredo Massieu #2
Borough: Colonia Magallanes
Work: (744) 485-6116
Mobile: 044-744-124-8683
Home: (744) 484-8788
Email: matadamashn@hotmail.com

Dr. Alejandro Reyes Rosas
Hospital del Pacifico,
Calle Fraile y Nao No. 4,
6th Floor, Room 606
Fraccionamiento La Bocana
Acapulco, Guerrero
Tel/Fax: (744) 488-1151 (office)
487-7180 (hospital)
482-9580 (home)
Mobile: 044-744-421-5317
Email: hanna_luna@hotmail.com

GASTROENTEROLOGISTS

Dr. Rafael Aguirre
General & Laparoscopic Surgery,
Gastroenterology
Address: Calle Nao #4

Borough: Colonia La Bocana
Work: (744) 488-1163
Fax: (744) 488-1160
Home: (744) 446-6616
Mobile: 044-744-449-2347
Email: raguri@prodigy.net.com

GENERAL MEDICINE

Dr. José Alfredo Leñero España
Hotel Copacabana
Tabachines 2 y 3
Fraccionamiento Club Deportivo
Acapulco, Guerrero
Tel: (744) 484-5556/1283

Dr. Alfonso H. Luz
General Medicine
Address: Calle Río Copala #21
Borough: Colonia Unidad
Habitacional Vicente Guerrero 2000
Work: (744) 466-9152
Home: (744) 462-1342
Mobile: 044-744-401-9178
Email: halfonso90@hotmail.com

GYNECOLOGISTS

Dr. José Silva
Obstetrics & Gynecology
Address: Calle Wilfredo Massieu #2
Office 204
Borough: Colonia Magallanes
Work: (744) 485-3699
Fax: (744) 485-6653
Home: (744) 483-5310
Mobile: 044-744-101-0343
Email: tirimacuaro@hotmail.com

INTERNIST

Dr. Carlos Galindo
Internal Medicine
Address: 2a. Calle Cristobal Colón #1623,
Office 102
Borough: Fraccionamiento Magallanes

Work: (744) 486-1515
Home: (744) 446-0719
Mobile: 044-744-449-0355
Email: galindo_md@hotmail.com

Dr. Norberto Matadamas
Internal Medicine, Cardiology
Address: Calle Wilfredo Massieu #2
Borough: Colonia Magallanes
Work: (744) 485-6116
Mobile: 044-744-124-8683
Home: (744) 484-8788
Email: matadamashn@hotmail.com

Dr. Alejandro Reyes
Internal Medicine, Cardiology &
Interventional Cardiology
Address: Calle Nao #4
Work/Fax: (744) 488-1151
Mobile: 044-744-421-5317
Email: hanna_luna@hotmail.com

OBSTETRICIANS

Dr. José Silva
Obstetrics & Gynecology
Address: Calle Wilfredo Massieu #2,
Office 204
Borough: Colonia Magallanes
Work: (744) 485-3699
Fax: (744) 485-6653
Home: (744) 483-5310
Mobile: 044-744-101-0343
Email: tirimacuaro@hotmail.com

ORTHOPEDIST

Dr. Ramon J. Ayerdi
Orthopedics/Traumatology
Address: Calle Vasco Nuñez de Balboa #1003,
Suite 204
Borough: Colonia Hornos
Work: (744) 486-5080
Home: (744) 483-4835
Mobile: 044-744-449-7853
Email: ram_jav@hotmail.com

PEDIATRICIANS

Dr. Gustavo Leyva
Pediatrics
Address: Calle Vasco Nuñez de Balboa #1003,
Office 206
Borough: Colonia Hornos
Work: (744) 486-5049
Home: (744) 487-7105
Mobile: 044-744-503-9927
Email: gusleyva30@hotmail.com

SURGEONS

Dr. Rafael Aguirre
General & Laparoscopic Surgery,
Gastroenterology
Address: Calle Nao #4
Borough: Colonia La Bocana
Work: (744) 488-1163
Fax: (744) 488-1160
Home: (744) 446-6616
Mobile: 044-744-449-2347
Email: raguri@prodigy.net.com

TRAUMATOLOGISTS

Dr. Ramon J. Ayerdi
Orthopedics/Traumatology
Address: Calle Vasco Nuñez de Balboa #1003,
Suite 204
Borough: Colonia Hornos
Work: (744) 486-5080
Home: (744) 483-4835
Mobile: 044-744-449-7853
Email: ram_jav@hotmail.com

HOSPITALS

Cruz Roja de Acapulco
Medical Area Costa Azul
Andrea Doria 1
Col. Costa Azul
Acapulco, Guerrero
Tel: (744) 481-3385 / 481-3880

Hospital Centro Médico
José Valdez Arévalo no. 620
Esq. Av. Cuauhtémoc. 3er. Piso
Acapulco, Guerrero
Tel: (744) 482-4692 / 4694 / 4693 / 1236,
483-2054
Fax: (744) 483-2724

Hospital Farallón
Av. Farallón No. 1, Lote 47
Fracc. La Garita
Acapulco, Guerrero
Tel: (744) 488-1557
Emergencies: (744) 469-9060

Hospital General Cd. Renacimiento
Ave. Juan R. Escudero (no street number)
Col. Renacimiento
Acapulco, Guerrero
Tel: (744) 441-4937 / 5621

Hospital General de Acapulco
Ave. Ruiz Cortines 128
Fracc. Alta Progreso
Acapulco, Guerrero
Tel: (744) 445-6608 / 5877

Hospital Magallanes
Address: Calle Wilfredo Massieu,
#2 (corner of Calle A. Amezquita)
Borough: Fraccionamiento Magallanes
Notable Landmarks:
Near "La Gran Plaza" Shopping Mall
Main Phone #: (744) 485-6544, 485-6594,
485-6596, 485-6597
Fax Phone #: (744) 485-6653

Hospital Naval de Acapulco
XVIII Zona Naval Militar
Ave. Costera Miguel Alemán No. 1
Col. Icacos
Acapulco, Guerrero
Tel: (744) 484-7053

Hospital Privado Magallanes
Calle Wilfrido Massieu 2
Fraccionamiento Magallanes
Acapulco, Guerrero
Tel: (744) 469-0270
Emergencies: ext. 104
Hospitalization: ext. 112

Hospital Santa Lucia
Vasco Nuñez de Balboa 1003
corner with J.R. Carrillo
Fraccionamiento Hornos
Acapulco, Guerrero
Tel: (744) 486-3358 / 3603

Medical Area Diamante
Blvd de las Naciones (no street number)
Col. Plan de los Amates
Acapulco, Guerrero
Tel: (744) 442-4883

Sanatorio Sagrado Corazón de Jesús
Calzada Pie de la Cuesta, lote 88-A
Fraccionamiento Mozimba
Acapulco, Guerrero
Tel: (744) 446-0642
admon@sanatoriosagradocorazon.com

Star Médica – Hospital del Pacifico
Address: Calle Nao #4
(Corner of Calle Fraile)
Borough: Fraccionamiento La Bocana,
Central Tourist Zone
Notable Landmarks:
"Plaza Bahia" Shopping Mall
and the "Cristo Rey" Church
Main Phone #: (744) 487-7180, 487-7161,
487-7308
Fax Phone #: (744) 485-2343

AGUASCALIENTES

HOSPITALS

Hospital Central Medico
Quirurgica Republica de Peru 102,
Fracc. Las Americas.
Aguascalientes, Aguascalientes
Tel: 01 (449) 910 6120
Emergencies: 24 hours

Hospital Miguel Hidalgo
Galeana 465,
Zona Centro Aguascalientes,
Aguascalientes
Tel: 01 (449) 994 6720 / (449) 915 8717
Emergencies: 24 hours

AGUA PRIETA

GENERAL MEDICINE

Dr. Heberto Molina Freaner,
Calle 2 y 3 Av. 4 No. 265
Phone: (633) 8-19-80

Dr. Daniel Rodarte de la Torre,
Calle 6 y Av. 20
Phone: (633) 8-06-40

HOSPITAL

Hospital Latinoamericano,
Calle 13 Av. 22 # 1280
Phone: (633) 8-31-92; 8-30-54 & 8-32- 44

AJIJIC
(ALSO SEE CHAPALA & GUADALAJARA)

HOSPITAL

Clínica Ajijic
Address: Carretera Oriente #33
(corner of Javier Mina)
Borough: Ajijic, Notable Landmarks:
Near Farmacia Guadalajara
Main Phone #: (376) 766-0662
Fax Phone #: (376) 766-0500
Email: ajijichospitalcenter@prodigy.net

AKUMAL

GENERAL MEDICINE

Dr. Nestor Mendoza
Address: Plaza "Ukana I" Local 24, Akumal
Work: (984) 875-9393
Fax: (984) 879-4040
Mobile: 044-984-806-4616
Email: dr_nestor_akumal@hotmail.com

ALAMOS

GENERAL MEDICINE

Dr. Joaquin Navarro Quijada,
General Medicine
Calle Juarez #4
Colonia Centro
Alamos, Sonora,
Phone: (647) 428-0310,
Fax: (647) 428-0398
Cel: (647) 482 1060
E-Mail: jnqalamos@hotmail.com

HOSPITALS

Hospital Basico de Alamos
Calle Madero
Prolongación Carretera Alamos-Sonora
Colonia Las Palmas
Alamos, Sonora,
Phone: (647) 428-0225, (647) 428-0226
E-Mail: saludhga@hotmail.com

BAHIA DE BANDERAS

HOSPITALS – PRIVATE

Hospital San Javier Riviera
Paseo de Los Cocoteros 55
Fracc. Nautico Turistico
Nuevo Vallarta
Bahia de Banderas, Nayarit
Tel. & Fax: (322) 226-8180 / 8181

HOSPITALS – PUBLIC

Hospital General "San Francisco"
Africa and China (no street number)
San Francisco
Bahía de Banderas, Nayarit
Tel. & Fax: (311) 258-4077 / 4229

CABO SAN LUCAS
(ALSO SEE SAN JOSE DEL CABO)

AMBULANCES

Medcare Ambulance Services
Matamoros y Niños Héroes
Colonia Centro, Cabo San Lucas,
Baja California Sur
Tel: (624) 143-4020
Fax: (624) 105-0176

DECOMPRESSION CHAMBER

Cruz Roja
Carretera Todos Santos Km. 121
Colonia Ejidal
Cabo San Lucas,
Tel: (624) 143-3300 / 7869
Fax: (624) 105-1500

Hospital de Especialidades
López Mateos (no street number),
between Leona Vicario y Morelos
Col. Ejidal
Cabo San Lucas
Tel: (624) 143-3666

DENTISTS

Dr. Roberto J. Altamira
Blvd. Lázaro Cárdenas
Edificio Pioneros Local 4
Cabo San Lucas,
Baja California Sur
Tel: (624) 143-0579
Fax: (624) 143-3340
Cell: (624) 355-4292
E-mail: bajadent@yahoo.com

Dra. Lorena de Ita Mejía
Dentistas Especialistas
Boulevard Lázaro Cárdenas
Edificio Coral,
across the street from McDonald's
Cabo San Lucas,
Baja California Sur
Tel: (624) 143-2299 / 4420 / 9994
E-mail:
dentistasespecabo@prodigy.net.mx

DERMATOLOGISTS

Dra. María del Carmen Ocampo
Hospital de Especialidades
López Mateos (no street number)
entre Leona Vicario y Morelos

Col. Ejidal, Cabo San Lucas,
Baja California Sur
Tel: (624) 143-3914

EMERGENCY MEDICINE

Dr. Alejandro Avalos
Emergency Medicine,
Orthopedics/Traumatology
Address: Avenida López Mateos
(at the corner of L. Vícario)
Borough: Colonia Ejidal
City: Cabo San Lucas
Work: (624) 143-7777, 143-2919
Fax: (624) 143-5457
Home: (624) 143-6567
Mobile: 044-624-147-0911
Email: direccion@bmr.com.mx,
bmr1@prodigy.net.mx

INTERNISTS

Dr. Pedro Alfonso Nájar Castañeda
Hospital de Especialidades
López Mateos
(between Leona Vicario y Morelos),
Colonia Ejidal, Cabo San Lucas,
Tel: (624)143-1218 / 2686
Cell: (624) 147-5919
Dr. Miguel Tolosa
Internal Medicine
Address: Avenida López Mateos
(at the corner of Calle Leona Vícario)
Borough: Colonia Ejidal
City: Cabo San Lucas
Work: (624) 143-7766, 143-7777, 143-3914
Fax: (624) 143-5407
Mobile: 044-624-122-0999
Email: migueltolosa.csnl@hotmail.com

OBSTETRICIANS/ GYNECOLOGISTS

Dr. Jorge Martín Niebla
Hospital de Especialidades

López Mateos (between Leona Vicario y
Morelos)
Colonia Ejidal, Cabo San Lucas,
Baja California Sur
Tel: (624) 143-2919 / 7777
Cell: (624) 141-6028

ORTHOPEDISTS

Dr. Alejandro Ávalos
Emergency Medicine,
Orthopedics/Traumatology
Hospital de Especialidades
López Mateos
(between Leona Vicario y Morelos)
Colonia Ejidal, Cabo San Lucas,
Baja California Sur
Tel: (624) 143-7777, (624) 143-2919 / 3914
Home: (624) 143-6567
Cell: (624) 147-0911
Email: direccion@bmr.com.mx,
bmr1@prodigy.net.mx

Dr. Gerardo Mangino
Orthopedics, Joint Replacement
Carretera Transpeninsular, Km 6.3
Tel: 624 104.39.11 or 12
Cell 1 624.183.73.89
info@caboorthopaedics.com

Dr. James McAllister
Orthopedics/Traumatology
Address: Calle Pescador, (no street number),
Office E-2 (near Camino Viejo a San José,
a couple blocks from the AmeriMed Hospital)
City: Cabo San Lucas
Work: (624) 143-5404, 143-7758
Fax: (624) 143-7758
Home: (624) 144-3569
Mobile: 044-624-141-6176
Email: footsmd@yahoo.com

Dr. Javier Escamilla Penagos
Orthopedics/Traumatology
Ave. Paseo de la Gaviota Esq.
con Blvd. Lazaro Cardenas
Dptos. el Dorado

Col. El Medano, Cabo San Lucas,
Baja California Sur
Tel: 6241051235

PEDIATRICIAN

Dr. Jorge Rafael Castro
Address: Avenida López Mateos
(between Morelos and Leona Vícario)
Borough: Colonia Ejidal
City: Cabo San Lucas
Work: (624) 143-3914
Home: (624) 173-4884
Mobile: 044-624-150-3092
Email: drjrtigger@prodigy.net.mx

SURGEON

Dr. Alejandro Ávalos L.
Hospital de Especialidades
López Mateos
(between Leona Vicario y Morelos)
Colonia Ejidal, Cabo San Lucas,
Baja California Sur
Tel: (624) 143-2919 / 3914
Cell: (624) 147-0911

Dr. Gerardo Garcia
General surgery, laproscopic and
bariatric surgery
Amerimed Hospital
Paseo de las Misiones at Careterra Transp,
624 158 3933

Dr. Felix Porras
Av. Pescador (no street number), E-1
Col. El Médano
Cabo San Lucas
fporras@prodigy.net.mx
624-183-3547
Cell: 624-147-5263

TRAUMATOLOGY

Dr. Alejandro Avalos
Emergency Medicine, Orthopedics/
Traumatology

Address: Avenida López Mateos
(at the corner of L. Vícario)
Borough: Colonia Ejidal, Cabo San Lucas
Work: (624) 143-7777, 143-2919
Fax: (624) 143-5457
Home: (624) 143-6567
Mobile: 044-624-147-0911
Email: direccion@bmr.com.mx,
bmr1@prodigy.net.mx

Dr. James McAllister
Orthopedics/Traumatology
Address: Calle Pescador, no street number, Office E-2 (near Camino Viejo a San José,
a couple blocks from the AmeriMed Hospital)
City: Cabo San Lucas
Work: (624) 143-5404, 143-7758
Fax: (624) 143-7758
Home: (624) 144-3569
Mobile: 044-624-141-6176
Email: footsmd@yahoo.com

HOSPITALS

Amerimed
Address: Boulevard Lázaro Cárdenas,
no street number (corner of Paseo de
la Marina) Pioneros Building 1
Borough: Colonia Medano
Notable Landmarks: Near McDonald's at entrance to town from airport
Main Phone/Fax #: (624) 143-9670, 143-9672,
143-9673 (request fax tone)

Balboa Hospital Los Cabos
Blvd. Lázaro Cárdenas 911
(between Paseo Gaviotas y Libramiento)
Cabo San Lucas,
Tel: (624) 143-5911

Centro Médico Cabo
Dr. Andrés Flores Gomez
Prolongación Juan Álvarez
(no street number)
Col. Arenal
Cabo San Lucas
Tel: 143-9727, 143-9728, 143-9729
Fax:143-1583

Centro Médico Cabo San Lucas
Prolongación Juan Álvarez
(no street number)
Col. El Arenal Libramiento Bordo
Cabo San Lucas
Tel: (624) 143-9727 / 9729
Cell: (624) 141-6010
Emergency number: (624) 143-1022
Fax: (624) 143-1583

Hospital de Especialidades
Address: Corner of Avenida López Mateos and
L. Vícario, (no street number)
Borough: Colonia Ejidal
Main Phone #: (624) 143-7777, 143-2919
Fax Phone #: (624) 143-5407
Emergency Phone #: (624) 144-3434

Northwest Medical
Pescador (no street number)
(Camino Viejo a San José)
Colonia El Médano (behind City Club store)
Cabo San Lucas, Baja California Sur
Tel: (624) 143-5404
Fax: (624) 143-7758
Cell: (624) 147-5263

CAMPECHE

HOSPITALS - PRIVATE

Clínica Campeche
Av. Central No. 65,
Col. Santa Ana,
phone: 811-0090 or 816-5612

Hospital Dr. Manuel Campos
Av. Blvd. (no street number),
Entre 14 Y 16,
phone: 816-5573

CANCUN

CARDIOLOGISTS

Dr. Gustavo Lopez Nava
Galenia Hospital
Av. Tulum, Lote 1
SM 12, MZ 1
Cancún, Quintana Roo
Tel: (998) 891-5200, ext. 204
Nextel: (998) 185-4614
Hours: 9-14 and 17 - 21

Dra. Carmen Saldivar
Internal Medicine, Electrodiagnostic
Cardiology
Address: Avenida Bonampak,
Lote #7, SM 10, Mza. 2
Work: (998) 881-3738, 881-3739
Fax: (998) 881-3737
Mobile: 044-998-874-3513
Email: carmen.saldivar@hospiten.com

Dr. Miguel Angel Yáñez
Galenia Hospital
Av. Tulum, Lote 1
SM 12, MZ 1
Cancún, Quintana Roo
Tel: (998) 891-5200 ext. 204
Cell: (998) 845-4427
Hours: 11:40-15

Dra. Carmen Zaldivar
Hospiten Hospital
Av. Bonampak, Lote 7
SM 10, MZ 2
Cancún, Quintana Roo
Tel: (998) 881-3700 / 3738 / 3739
Nextel: (998) 112-9777

COLPOSCOPY

Dra. Linda Velasco
Obstetrics/Gynecology, Colposcopy
Address: Avenida La Costa #120
Work: (998) 887-8708, 887-1100
Mobile: (044) 998-734-8236
Email: linda.velasco@hotmail.com

EAR, NOSE & THROAT

Dr. J. Federico Williamson
Address: Avenida Bonampak Lote #7,
SM 10 Mza. 2
Work: (998) 881-3738, 881-3739
Fax: (998) 881-3737
Mobile: 044-998-845-1052
Email: fwilliamson@hospiten.com

DENTISTS

Dr. Joaquín Berron
Dentaris Odontología Integral,
Av. Tulum 232-7C, Sm 4,
phone: 887-3979 or
892-1099 emergencies
Nextel – 282-3091)
www.dentaris.com.mx

Dr. Luis Armando Camacho Jimenez
Av. La Luna Numero 21
Supermanzana 43
Phone: 206-1826 & 206-2595
armadental@hotmail.com

Interdental (several dentists)
Calle Cereza 9 Supermanzana 2-A
Phone: 884-8379
www.inter-dental.com

Dra. Marisela Morales
Blvd. Kukulcan Km. 12.5
Centro Empresarial I-4
Zona Hotelera
Cancun, Quintana Roo
Tel: (998) 176-8084
Emergencies Cell: (998) 186-0560

Dr. Raúl Vargas Fonseca
Calle Robalo 39-3, SM 3
Cancún, Quintana Roo
Tel: (998) 884-3390
Emergencies Cell:(998) 120-1018 / 168-8652

Dr. José Alfredo Zuñiga Portilla
Calle Sierra 14, SM 3
Cancún, Quintana Roo
Tel: (998) 884-7731 / 7642
Emergencies Cell:(998) 845-7119

DIVING MEDICINE

Dr. César Soto
General Medicine, Diving Medicine,
Hyperbaric Medicine
Address: Alcatraces Lote #44,
SM 22, Mza. 10
(half block from the Palapas Park)
Borough: Colonia Centro
Work: (998) 892-7680
Mobile: 044-998-105-7791
Email: drcesarsoto@yahoo.com.mx

ENDOCRINOLOGY

Dr. Héctor R. Rivero
Pediatrics, Endocrinology
Address: Avenida Nichupté Lote #22,
SM 19, Mza. 2 (at the corner of Xpuhil),
in the Pabellón Caribe Building
Work: (998) 898-1394
Fax: (998) 898-1395
Pager: 01-800-835-2350
PIN #: 9988457490
Mobile: 044-998-845-7490
Email: hrriveroe@hotmail.com

GENERAL MEDICINE

Dr. César Soto
General Medicine, Diving Medicine,
Hyperbaric Medicine
Address: Alcatraces Lote #44,
SM 22, Mza. 10 (half block from the

Palapas Park)
Borough: Colonia Centro
Work: (998) 892-7680
Mobile: 044-998-105-7791
Email: drcesarsoto@yahoo.com.mx

HYPERBARIC MEDICINE

Dr. César Soto
General Medicine, Diving Medicine, Hyperbaric
Medicine
Address: Alcatraces Lote #44,
SM 22, Mza. 10
(half block from the Palapas Park)
Borough: Colonia Centro
Work: (998) 892-7680
Mobile: 044-998-105-7791
Email: drcesarsoto@yahoo.com.mx

GASTRIC ENDOSCOPY

Dr. Luis A. Guillermo
General Surgery, Gastric Endoscopy,
Laparoscopy
Address: Avenida Bonampak,
Lote #7, SM 10, Mza. 2
Work: (998) 881-3738, 881-3739
Fax: (998) 881-3737
Mobile: 044-998-845-6631
Email: lguillermo@hospiten.com

GYNECOLOGISTS

Dr. Jesús Rodríguez
Obstetrics/Gynecology
Address: Avenida Nichupté Lote #22,
SM 19, Mza. 2, Office 213
(at the corner of Xpuhil),
in the Pabellón Caribe Building
Work: (998) 898-0565
Mobile: 044-998-845-3962
Email: drjesusrc@prodigy.net.mx

Dra. Linda Velasco
Obstetrics/Gynecology, Colposcopy
Address: Avenida La Costa #120

Work: (998) 887-8708, 887-1100
Mobile: (044) 998-734-8236
Email: linda.velasco@hotmail.com

INTERNIST

Dr. Carlos M. Buenfil
Internal Medicine, Pulmonology,
Interventional Bronchology
Address: Calle Centella #4, SM 18,
Mza. 4 (Near Avenida Labna)
Work: (998) 887-3800
Home: (998) 884-3563
Mobile: 044-998-116-1211
Email: carlosbuenfil@hotmail.com

Dr. William H. Navarrete
Internal Medicine
Address: Avenida Bonampak,
Lote #7, SM 10, Mza. 2
Work: (998) 881-3738, 881-3739
Fax: (998) 881-3737
Mobile: 044-998-100-1693
Email: wnavarrete@hospiten.com

Dra. Carmen Saldivar
Internal Medicine, Electrodiagnostic
Cardiology
Address: Avenida Bonampak
Lote #7, SM 10, Mza. 2
Work: (998) 881-3738, 881-3739
Fax: (998) 881-3737
Mobile: 044-998-874-3513
Email: carmen.saldivar@hospiten.com

LAPARASCOPY

Dr. Luis A. Guillermo
General Surgery, Gastric Endoscopy,
Laparoscopy
Address: Avenida Bonampak,
Lote #7, SM 10, Mza. 2
Work: (998) 881-3738, 881-3739
Fax: (998) 881-3737
Mobile: 044-998-845-6631
Email: lguillermo@hospiten.com

NEONATOLOGY

Dra. Rosa E. Olivares
Pediatrics & Neonatology
Address: Avenida Nichupté Lote #22,
SM 19, Mza. 2 (at the corner of Xpuhil),
in the Pabellón Caribe Building
Work: (998) 872-3208
Mobile: 044-998-845-4644
Email: rolitanto@hotmail.com

OBSTETRICIANS

Dr. Jesús Rodríguez
Obstetrics/Gynecology
Address: Avenida Nichupté Lote #22,
SM 19, Mza. 2, Office 213
(at the corner of Xpuhil),
in the Pabellón Caribe Building
Work: (998) 898-0565
Mobile: 044-998-845-3962
Email: drjesusrc@prodigy.net.mx

Dra. Linda Velasco
Obstetrics/Gynecology, Colposcopy
Address: Avenida La Costa #120
Work: (998) 887-8708, 887-1100
Mobile: (044) 998-734-8236
Email: linda.velasco@hotmail.com

PEDIATRICIANS

Dra. Elena Carmona
Pediatrics
Address: Avenida Nichupté Lote #22,
SM 19, Mza. 2, Office 213
(at the corner of Xpuhil),
in the Pabellón Caribe Building
Work: (998) 898-0568
Home: (998) 889-9070
Mobile: 044-998-845-8482
Email: elena_carmona@hotmail.com

Dra. Rosa E. Olivares
Pediatrics & Neonatology
Address: Avenida Nichupté Lote #22,

SM 19, Mza. 2
(at the corner of Xpuhil),
in the Pabellón Caribe Building
Work: (998) 872-3208
Mobile: 044-998-845-4644
Email: rolitanto@hotmail.com

Dr. Héctor R. Rivero
Pediatrics, Endocrinology
Address: Avenida Nichupté Lote #22,
SM 19, Mza. 2
(at the corner of Xpuhil),
in the Pabellón Caribe Building
Work: (998) 898-1394
Fax: (998) 898-1395
Pager: 01-800-835-2350,
PIN #: 9988457490
Mobile: 044-998-845-7490
Email: hrriveroe@hotmail.com

PSYCHIATRY

Dr. Enrique Barrales Islas
Bonampak 28 Interior 18
Supermanzana 4
Phone: 892-4089
drbarrales@hotmail.com

PULMONOLOGY

Dr. Carlos M. Buenfil
Internal Medicine, Pulmonology,
Interventional Bronchology
Address: Calle Centella #4,
SM 18, Mza. 4 (Near Avenida Labna)
Work: (998) 887-3800
Home: (998) 884-3563
Mobile: 044-998-116-1211
Email: carlosbuenfil@hotmail.com

SURGEON

Dr. Luis A. Guillermo
General Surgery, Gastric Endoscopy,
Laparoscopy
Address: Avenida Bonampak,

Lote #7, SM 10, Mza. 2
Work: (998) 881-3738, 881-3739
Fax: (998) 881-3737
Mobile: 044-998-845-6631
Email: lguillermo@hospiten.com

HOSPITALS - PRIVATE

Clinica Quirurgica del Sur
Avenida Lopez Portillo Manzana 37,
Lotes 2 y 3 Supermanzana 59
Unidad Morelos
Phone: 886-7636 & 843-5454
http://www.quirurgicadelsur.com/

Clinica Sobrino
Manzana Q, Lote 13, Supermanzana 63
Phone: 884-2516
clinicasobrino@yahoo.com.mx

Hiperbarica Cancún
Hyperbaric Chamber Facility
Facility Certification #: 021.05-A000237
Address: Alcatraces Lote #44,
SM 22, Mza. 10
(half block from the Palapas)
Borough: Colonia Centro
Main/Fax Phone #: (998) 892-7680

Hospital Americano
Retorno Viento No. 15
SM 4, MZ 22
Cancún, Quintana Roo
Tel: (998) 884-6133 / 287-8022
Fax: (998) 884-6425
24 hr Emergency and Intensive therapy:
Tel: (998) 884-6068

Hospital Amerimed
Av. Tulum Sur 260
SM 7, MZ 4, 5 y 9
Cancún, Quintana Roo
Tel & Fax: (998) 881-3400
http://www.amerimedcancun.com/

Hospital Galenia
Av. Tulum, Lote 1
SM 12, MZ 1

Fracc. Sta Maria Siké
Cancún, Quintana Roo
Tel: (998) 891-5200
www.hospitalgalenia.com

Hospital Hospiten
Av. Bonampak, Lote 7
SM 10, MZ 2
Cancún, Quintana Roo
Tel: (998) 881-3700 / 3738 / 3739
Emergencies: 01-800-900-9009
http://www.hospiten.com/

Hospital Presbiteriano
Region 76 Manzana 46 Lote 1
Colonia Francisco Villa
Phone: 880-2082 & 880-4006
hospipres@prodigy.net.mx

HOSPITALS - PUBLIC

Hospital General
Andador 5
SM 65, entre calle 12 X 13
Cancún, Quintana Roo
Tel: (998) 884-2967 / 2666

CHAPALA
ALSO SEE AJIJIC AND GUADALAJARA

CARDIOLOGY

Dr. Salvador E. Flores
Internal Medicine, Cardiology, Interventional
Cardiology, Sports Medicine
Chapala Address: Carretera Oriente #33
Borough: Colonia Centro
Chapala Work: (376) 766-0662, 766-0500
Guadalajara Address: Tarascos #3422
Borough: Fraccionamiento Monraz
Guadalajara Work: (33) 3813-0540,
3813-0547
Home: 01-33-3641-9021

Mobile: 01-33-3105-2773
Pager: 01-33-1515-1111, PIN# 3012

GENERAL MEDICINE

Dr. Alfredo Rodríguez
Address: Carretera Ote. #33
Borough: Colonia Centro
Work: (376) 766-0662
Fax: (376) 766-0500
Mobile: 044-33-3106-1770
Email: drarodriguez12@hotmail.com

INTERNISTS

Dr. Salvador E. Flores
Internal Medicine, Cardiology,
Interventional Cardiology, Sports Medicine
Chapala Address: Carretera Oriente #33
Borough: Colonia Centro
Chapala Work: (376) 766-0662, 766-0500
Guadalajara Address: Tarascos #3422
Borough: Fraccionamiento Monraz
Guadalajara Work: (33) 3813-0540,
3813-0547
Home: 01-33-3641-9021
Mobile: 01-33-3105-2773
Pager: 01-33-1515-1111, PIN# 3012

Dr. Carlos García
Internal Medicine
Address: 79G Hidalgo
Borough: Riberas del Pilar
Work/Fax: (376) 765-4805
Mobile: 01-33-3129-7705
Email: gardica@yahoo.com

ORTHOPEDICIANS

Dr. Jesús Campos
Orthopedics/Traumatology
Address: Carretera Oriente #33
Borough: Colonia Centro
Work/fax: (376) 766-0500, 766-0662
Home: (33) 3832-2223
Mobile: 044-33-3106-4180

Pager: (33) 3678-4300, PIN# 1581
Email: jesus_campos@doctor.com

TRAUMATOLOGISTS

Dr. Jesús Campos
Orthopedics/Traumatology
Address: Carretera Oriente #33
Borough: Colonia Centro
Work/fax: (376) 766-0500, 766-0662
Home: (33) 3832-2223
Mobile: 044-33-3106-4180
Pager: (33) 3678-4300, PIN# 1581
Email: jesus_campos@doctor.com

HOSPITAL

Clinica Maskaras
Calle Hidalgo #79-G
(on the Chapala-Jocotepec Highway)
Riberas del Pilar
Tel: (376) 765-4805
Tel/Fax: (376) 765-4838
Farmacy: (376) 765-5827
Open: 24 hours

CHETUMAL

HOSPITAL

Hospital General de Chetumal
Av. Andrés Quintana Roo 399
Colonia Taxistas
(next to Escuela Tecnológico)
Chetumal, Quintana Roo
Tel: (983) 832-1953 / 1977 / 1932

CHIAPA DE CORZO

HOSPITALS

Centro de Salud
Calle Julián Grajales
corner with Calle Iturbide
Barrio de San Pedro
Chiapa de Corzo, Chiapas
Tel: (961) 616-0205

Cruz Roja
Rivera Namdanbua
Carretera Internacional Km. 14.5
Libramiento Norte
Chiapa de Corzo, Chiapas
Tel: (961) 616-1900

CHIHUAHUA

HOSPITALS

Centro Médico de Especialidades
16 de Septiembre No. 24
Chilpancingo, Guerrero
Tel: (747) 472-7730

Clínica Chilpancingo
Ave. Castrejón 17-A
Chilpancingo, Guerrero
Tel: (747) 472-7499

Clínica Hospital ISSSTE
Ave. Ruffo Figueroa s-n
Chilpancingo, Guerrero
Tels: (747) 472-0008 / 0424 / 3162

Cruz Roja
Ave. Juárez corner with Uruguay
Col. Centro
Chilpancingo, Guerrero
Tel: (747) 472-6562 / 6561

Hospital General
Dr. Raymundo Abarca Alarcón
Ave. Vicente Guerrero 45
Col. Centro
Chilpancingo, Guerrero
Tel: (747) 472-2031 / 0990

Hospital Privado Anáhuac
Ignacio Ramírez No.74
Chilpancingo, Guerrero
Tel: (747) 472-9505 / 471-1420

Sanatorio América
Altamirano 56
Chilpancingo, Guerrero
Tel: (747) 472-2976

Sanatorio Nuestra Señora del Carmen
Ave. Juarez # 53
Chilpancingo, Guerrero
Tel: (747) 472-2380

SDN Hospital Militar Regional
35 Zona Militar, Campo Militar 2
Hermenegildo Galeana 35a
Chilpancingo, Guerrero
Tel: (747) 472-9986 / 7536 / 2279

CHILPANCINGO

HOSPITALS

Centro Médico de Especialidades
16 de Septiembre No. 24
Chilpancingo, Guerrero
Tel: (747) 472-7730

Clínica Chilpancingo
Ave. Castrejón 17-A
Chilpancingo, Guerrero
Tel: (747) 472-7499

Clínica Hospital ISSSTE
Ave. Ruffo Figueroa s-n
Chilpancingo, Guerrero
Tels: (747) 472-0008 / 0424 / 3162

Cruz Roja
Ave. Juárez corner with Uruguay
Col. Centro
Chilpancingo, Guerrero
Tel: (747) 472-6562 / 6561

Hospital General
Dr. Raymundo Abarca Alarcón
Ave. Vicente Guerrero 45
Col. Centro
Chilpancingo, Guerrero
Tel: (747) 472-2031 / 0990

Hospital Privado Anáhuac
Ignacio Ramírez No.74
Chilpancingo, Guerrero
Tel: (747) 472-9505 / 471-1420

Sanatorio América
Altamirano 56
Chilpancingo, Guerrero
Tel: (747) 472-2976

Sanatorio Nuestra Señora del Carmen
Ave. Juarez # 53
Chilpancingo, Guerrero
Tel: (747) 472-2380

SDN Hospital Militar Regional
35 Zona Militar, Campo Militar 2
Hermenegildo Galeana 35a
Chilpancingo, Guerrero
Tel: (747) 472-9986 / 7536 / 2279

CIUDAD DEL CARMEN

HOSPITALS - PRIVATE

Central Quirúrgica Del Carmen
Calle 22, No. 188,
phone: 382-3468

Centro Medico Carmen
Calle 58, No. 51, Col. Fatima,
phone: 384-4300

Clínica De Especialidades Médicas
Del Carmen
Calle 42, No. 79, Aviacion,
phone: 382-6906, 382-9387, or 382-1867

Clínica Morelos
Calle 57, No. 1,
phone: 382-3942

Grupo San Miguel
Calle 50, No. 1, Col. Caleta,
phone: 384-1002 or 1003

HOSPITALS - PUBLIC

Cruz Roja (Mexican Red Cross)
Calle 56, (no street number),
Col. Centro, phone: 384-0447

CIUDAD ACUÑA

FAMILY MEDICINE

Dr. Bernardo De La Garza Hernandez,
Address: Hidalgo #1613

Specialties: Family Medicine & Obesity
Phone: 772-6663
U.S. Phone: 830-488-3421

GYNECOLOGISTS

Dr. Javier Benitez Coria,
Address: Manuel Acufia #365
Specialty: Gynecologist
Phone: 888-0746

Dr. Oscar Faz Hipolito,
Address: 16 de Septiembre #295
Specialty: Gynecologist
Phone: 772-2071

CIUDAD JUAREZ

ALLERGY/ IMMUNOLOGY

Dr. Ruben Villegas Heredia
Address: 1913 Ignacio Mejia St
Ciudad Juarez
Phone: 656 614-7492

CARDIOLOGISTS

Dr. Luis Rodolfo Flores Montano
Address: De Las Americas 201
Ciudad Juarez
Phone: 656 613-6554

DENTISTS

Dr. Ruben Escobar Prieto
Address: Constitucion 383
Col. Centro, Ciudad Juarez
Phone: 656 612-0259, 614-0767

Dr. Ernesto Alonso Moran
Address: Blvd. Tomas Fernandez 1803 Int. 2
Phone: 616-1731, (915) 613-5233

Dr. Jorge Ramos Burgos
Address: Av. Malecon 200
Phone: 656 612-5714

DERMATOLOGISTS

Dr. Maria Griselda Alcaraz
Address: Ave. Lopez Mateos 1364 Sur
Phone: 613-2121, 613-2154, 613-2081

EAR, NOSE & THROAT

Dr. Ignacio Peraldi Rios
Address: Paseo De La Victoria 4370, Int. 821
Phone: 616-7717, 611-2727

GENERAL MEDICINE

Dr. Mark R. Reeves
General Medicine
Address: Avenida Las Americas #722
Borough: Colonia Margaritas
U.S. Work: +1-915-581-3176
Mexico Work: (656) 617-0461
U.S. Fax: +1-915-584-6759
U.S. Mobile: +1-915-549-2820
Email: mrrmdny@aol.com

GASTROENTEROLOGY

Dr. Felipe Fornelli Lafon
Address: Ave. de las Americas 201
int. 104-B
Phone: 613-9945

Dr. Jorge Blake Siemsen
Address: Campos Eliseos 9371
Phone: 618-0982, 227-1980

GYNECOLOGISTS

Dr. Joaquin Esquivel Anaya
Address: Av. Lopez Mateos 248
Phone: 613-6152,
In the U.S. (915-239-0362)

Dr. Jorge Rocha-López
Obstetrics & Gynecology
Address: Avenida Las Americas #722
Borough: Margaritas
Work: (656) 616-4245
Fax: (656) 619-7010
Mobile: 044-656-215-1521
Pager: (656) 629-0999, PIN # 100154
Email: drrocha@hotmail.com

OBSTETRICIAN

Dr. Jorge Rocha-López
Obstetrics & Gynecology
Address: Avenida Las Americas #722
Borough: Margaritas
Work: (656) 616-4245
Fax: (656) 619-7010
Mobile: 044-656-215-1521
Pager: (656) 629-0999, PIN # 100154
Email: drrocha@hotmail.com

ONCOLOGY

Dr. Enrique Silva Perez
Address: Pedro Rosales De Leon 7510
int. 220
Phone: 618-1558, 618-3564

OPHTHALMOLOGY

Dr. Francisco Berumen
Address: Av. de las Americas 555 Norte
Phone: 613-5250

ORTHOPEDICS

Dr. Roberto Moreno Razo
Address: Av. de las Americas 678 Norte
Phone: 616-2094

Dr. Carlos Montes
Orthopedics and Traumatology
Address: Calle Pedro Rosales de León #7510
Borough: Colonia Fuentes del Valle

Work/Fax: (656) 618-3707
Mobile: 044-656-191-0633
Email: carlo104@prodigy.net.mx

PEDIATRICIANS

Dr. Jorge Pérez-Lucio
Address: Calle Pedro S. Varela #3007
(at Avenida Las Americas and
Calle Lincoln)
Borough: Colonia La Playa
Work: (656) 616-2753, 616-1610
Fax: +1-915-581-3407 (U.S. number)
Pager: (656) 629-0999, PIN# 105498
Email: jorgepelucio@yahoo.com

PSYCHIATRY

Dr. Alejandro Ibarra Valdez
Address: Pedro Rosales De Leon 7510
int. 201
Phone: 618-4288

TRAUMATOLOGISTS

Dr. Carlos Montes
Orthopedics and Traumatology
Address: Calle Pedro Rosales de León #7510
Borough: Colonia Fuentes del Valle
Work/Fax: (656) 618-3707
Mobile: 044-656-191-0633
Email: carlo104@prodigy.net.mx

RADIOLOGY

Dra. Estela Moreno
Address: Av. de las Americas 678 Norte
Phone: 616-2094

RHEUMATOLOGY

Dra. Rosalinda Cruz
Address: intersection Lerdo and 16 de
Septiembre streets, int. 11
Phone: 612-4897

UROLOGY

Dr. Hector Calderon
Address: Av. de las Americas 201, int. 206
Phone: 613-0767

HOSPITALS

Hospital Poliplaza Médica
Address: Calle Pedro Rosales de León #7510
Borough: Colonia Fuentes del Valle
Main/Fax Phone #: (656) 623-6249
Website: www.polizplaza.com

CIUDAD MANTE

CARDIOLOGISTS

Dr. Jorge Antonio Aguirre Contreras,
Calle Guerrero #211 Ote,
Zona Centro
Office hours: 10 am to 2 pm & 7 pm to 8 pm
Tel: (831) 232-16 33
E-mail: drjorgeaguirre@hotmail.com
Specializing in: Cardiology
Universidad Nacional Autónoma de México
Forty-two years of experience.

GASTROENTEROLOGISTS

Dr. Leonardo Reyes Hernández,
Specializing in: Gastroenterology and surgery
Morelos #105 Sur, Zona Centro
Office hours: 9 am to 1 pm & 8 pm to 9:30 pm
Monday–Friday, 9 am to 2 Saturday
Tel: (831) 239-5312
Universidad Autónoma de Tamaulipas and Universidad Autónoma de Nuevo León.
Twenty-four years of experience.

GENERAL SURGEONS

Dr. Juan José García Zamudio,
Calle Guerrero #508-B, Zona Centro,
Office hours: 11 am to 5 pm
Tel & Fax: (831) 233-34 92
E-mail: myana1311@hotmail.com
Specializing in: General Surgery
Universidad de Guadalajara y
Universidad de Nuevo León
Twenty years of experience.

INTERNISTS

Dr. Severo Medina Martínez,
Specializing in: General Medicine
Calle Pedro J. Mendez #210 Nte. Interior,
Zona Centro
Office hours: 9 to 1 pm
Tel: (831) 232-1557
Universidad Nacional Autónoma de México
Thirty years of experience.

OPHTALMOLOGISTS

Dr. Carlos López Baca,
Calle Guerrero #118 Ote., Zona Centro
Office hours: 9 am to 1 pm and 8 pm to 9 pm
Tel: (831) 232-2997
E-mail: dr.carloslopezbaca@hotmail.com
Universidad Autónoma de Nuevo León
Fifteen years of experience.

ORTHOPEDICS/ TRAUMATOLOGISTS

Dr. Raúl Fernando Manrique Adame,
Specializing in: Orthopedics & Traumatology
Calle Guerrero # 118 Ote. Zona Centro
Office hours: 10 am to 1 pm & 5 pm to 8 pm
Monday–Friday, 10 pm to 1 pm Saturday
Tel & Fax: (831) 232-13 44
E-mail: raferman53@hotmail.com
Universidad Autónoma de San Luis Potosi
Thirty years of experience.

Dr. Rafael Martínez Castruita
Specializing in: Orthopedics & Traumatology
Calle Hidalgo No. 102 Sur,
Plaza Ramsal, Interior 7, Zona Centro
Office hours: 12 pm to 5 pm
Tel: (831) 23 2 86 35
Fax: (831) 23 4 01 50
E-mail: dr.rafaelmc@hotmail.com
Universidad Autónoma Nuevo León,
Centro Médico de Occidente, I.M.S.S.
Centro Médico del Noreste.
Twenty-two years of experience.

PEDIATRICIANS

Dr. Pastor Rosales Castellón,
Specializing in: Pediatrics & Gastroenterology
Calle Morelos No.105 Sur
Office hours: 10 am to 2 pm & 6 am to 9 pm
Monday–Saturday
Tel & Fax: (831) 23 2 10 96
E-mail: parc12@prodigy.net.mx
Universidad Veracruzana,
Hospital Infantil de México "Federico Gómez"
and Hospitales Infantiles en México.
Twenty years of experience.

REUMATOLOGIST

Dr. Lucas Sánchez Torres,
Calle Morelos #105 Sur
Office hours: 9 am to 2 pm & 3 pm to 8 pm
Monday–Friday, 9 am to 2 pm Saturday
Tel & Fax: (831) 234-3702
E-mail: drlusato@hotmail.com
Specializing in: rheumatology
Universidad Autónoma de Tamaulipas
Twenty-four years of experience.

HOSPITALS

Centro de Salud
Rio Mante 300, Zona Centro
Tel: (831) 232 12 96, 232 04 12,
232 5201 18

Hospital "de Praga"
Av. Juárez #501 Ote,
Zona Centro
Tel: 831-232-0200

Hospital General
Calle Sabino #300, Colonia Altavista
Tel: 831-233-8160

Instituto Mexicano del Seguro (IMSS)
Blvd. Luis Echeverría Alvarez y Obregón #300,
Zona Centro
Tel: 831-232-1244

CIUDAD OBREGON

ANESTHESIOLOGISTS

Dr. Javier Lopez Navarro
Anesthesiology
Centro Médico Sur Sonora
Calle Norte No. 749 Oriente
Cd. Obregon, Sonora,
Phone: (644) 415-0881, (644) 415-0044
Fax: 415-2640,
Cell: (644) 448-2354
E-mail: drlopezn@hotmail.com
drlopezn@cob-megared.net.mx

CARDIOLOGISTS

Dr. Gonzalo Gutierrez Robles
Cardiology
Clínica San Alfonso
Calle Coahuila #616 Sur
Colonia Centro
Ciudad Obregon, Sonora
Phone/Fax: (644) 417-0079,
(644) 412-1563

GASTROENTEROLOGIST

Dr. Armando Barreda Pesqueira
Gastroenterologist
Clinica La Purisima General Practice
Veracruz 621 norte General Surgery
Ciudad Obregon, Sonora,
Phone: (644) 415-1518, 414-8811
E-Mail: barredapar@hotmail.com

GENERAL PRACTICE / SURGERY

Dr. Armando Barreda Pesqueira
Clínica San José
No. Reelección 101 Oriente
Ciudad Obregón, Sonora
Tel: (644) 415-0202
Fax: (644) 413-1425
E-mail: barreda@gatelink.net

INTERNISTS

Dr. José Luís Rodríguez Martínez
California No. 153 Sur
Colonia Centro
Ciudad Obregón, Sonora
Tel. & Fax: (644) 413-4898

ONCOLOGIST

Dr. Pedro Adrian Gonzalez Rivera
Oncologist
Clínica San José,
No Reeleccion 101 Oriente
Ciudad Obregon, Sonora
Phone: (644) 415-0202
Cell (644) 408-9788

OPHTALMOLOGISTS

Dr. Raul Castro de la Cruz
Clínica San José,
No Reeleccion 101 Oriente
Colonia Centro, Ciudad Obregon, Sonora

Phone: (644) 415-0770
Fax: (644) 413-2814
E-Mail: raulcastro@opticamoderna.com

Dr. Guillermo Saviñon Plaza
Río Pánuco #713 poniente
Ciudad Obregon, Sonora,
Phone: (644) 413-4407,
fax 644/413-4404
E-Mail: cagsavignon@infocel.net.mx home
drsavinon@hotmail.com office

Dr. Jose Carlos Urrea Salazar
Calle 5 de Febrero #749
on the corner of Norte
Cd. Obregon, Sonora,
Phone: (644) 414-0992, ext. 146
Fax: (644) 415-2640

ORTHOPEDICS

Dr. Samuel B. Diaz Corral
California 153 Sur Traumatology
Ciudad Obregon, Sonora,
Phone: (644) 414-4802
E-mail: samuel_bernardo@hotmail.com

HOSPITALS

Centro Medico Sur Sonora
Calle Norte No.749 Oriente
Ciudad Obregón, Sonora
Tel: (644) 415-0409, 414-2428

Clinica San Jose
Calle No Reeleccion 101 oriente
Cd. Obregon, Sonora,
Phone: (644) 415-0202

Clinica Santa Margarita
Sinaloa No. 334 Norte
Colonia Centro
Ciudad Obregón, Sonora
Tel: (644) 414-3000 / 9266

Hospital General
Plutarco Elias Calles (no street number)

Cd. Obregon, Sonora,
Phone: (644) 417-3555, (644) 416-4009,
(644) 416-4322, (644) 416-4374
Fax: (644) 416-4635 ext. 123

Hospital San Jose
Coahuila No. 263 Sur
Ciudad Obregón, Sonora
Tel: (644) 415-0233 / 0243 / 0151 / 9570

Maternidad San Gerardo
Nainari No. 1155 Poniente
Ciudad Obregón, Sonora
Tel: (644) 414-7919 / 8290

CIUDAD VALLES

HOSPITAL

Hospital General de Ciudad Valles
Carretera México-Laredo Km. 7,
on the corner of Ángel Oliva, Col. Oxitipa
Ciudad Valles, San Luis Potosí,
Telephone (481) 381-3210
Fax (481) 381-3451 ext. 204

CIUDAD VICTORIA

DENTISTS

Dra. María Magdalena De Alba Rumenus
Calle Morelos Ote. #739,
Zona Centro
Office hours: 9 am to 5 pm, Monday–Friday
9 am to 1 pm Saturdays
Tel: (834) 31 2 80 64
Email: dradealba@hotmail.com

Dr. Ernesto Arnoldo Rodríguez Sánchez,
Specializing in: Endodontics
16 Matamoros y Morelos No. 212,
Zona Centro
Office hours: 7 am to 7 pm
Tel: (834) 31 2 71 89
Universidad Autónoma de Nuevo León
Nineteen years of experience.

Dr. Gustavo Adolfo Tirado Saldívar,
Specializing in: Orthodontics
Ave. Carrera Torres 14 No. 394-6 Ote.
Office hours: 9 am to 1 pm & 3:30 pm to 7 pm
Tel: (834) 31 6 95 74
Fax: (834) 31 5 16 00
Universidad Autónoma de Nuevo León,
Georgetown University, Washington D.C.
Twenty-seven years of experience.

Dr. José Manuel Tirado Saldívar,
Ave. Carrera Torres No. 405 Ote.
Office hours: 10 am to 1 pm & 4 pm to 7 pm
Tel: (834) 316 8914
Fax: (834) 315 1600
E-mail: jmtiradosal@hotmail.com
Universidad Autónoma de Nuevo León
Forty-three years of experience.

EAR, NOSE & THROAT

Dr. Pablo Alejandro Beltran Castro,
Specializing in: Otorhinolaryngology
12 y 13 Matamoros No. 514, Zona Centro
Office hours: 9 am to 1 pm & 4 pm to 8 pm
Monday–Friday
Tel & Fax: (834) 31 2 04 14
Email: pabc_53@hotmail.com
Universidad Autónoma de Tamaulipas and Universidad Autónoma de Nuevo León.
Twenty-six years of experience.

ENDOCRINOLOGIST

Dr. Alejandro Tirado Saldívar
Specializing in: Internal Medicine &
Endocrinology

Calle Gaspar de la Garza Sur #181-A,
Zona Centro
Office hours: 10 am to 1 pm & 4 pm to 7 pm
Monday–Friday, 10 am to 1 pm Saturdays
Tel y Fax: (834) 31 2 48 63
E-mail: dr_atirado@hotmail.com
Universidad Autónoma de Nuevo León,
St. Louis University Medical Center and
University of Maryland
Thirty-eight years of experience. 13

GASTROENTEROLOGISTS

Dr. Rafael Guevara García,
Specializing in: Gastroenterology and
Gastrointestinal Endoscopy
Calle 17 Guerrero y Bravo #409,
Zona Centro
Office hours: 10 am to 1 pm & 5 pm to 8 pm
Monday–Friday
Tel: (834) 3 15 11 37
E-mail: drguevara@prodigy.net.mx
Universidad Nacional Autonoma de Méxio and
Centro Medico Nacional Siglo XXI.
Twenty-one years of experience.

INTERNIST

Dr. Alejandro Tirado Saldívar
Specializing in: Internal Medicine &
Endocrinology
Calle Gaspar de la Garza Sur #181-A,
Zona Centro
Office hours: 10 am to 1 pm & 4 pm to 7 pm
Monday–Friday, 10 am to 1 pm Saturdays
Tel y Fax: (834) 31 2 48 63
E-mail: dr_atirado@hotmail.com
Universidad Autónoma de Nuevo León,
St. Louis University Medical Center and
University of Maryland
Thirty-eight years of experience. 13

PEDIATRICIANS

Dr. Manuel Garza Sanchez,
12 y 13 Aldama #504, Zona Centro
Office hours: 11 am to 1 pm & 4 pm to 8:30 pm
Monday–Friday, 11 am to 4 pm Saturdays
Tel: (834) 3 16 91 43
E-mail: manuel8343@prodigy.net.mx
Universidad Autonoma de Nuevo Leon and
Universidad Autonoma de Tamaulipas
Fifteen years of experience.

SURGEON

Dr. Hector Eduardo Diaz Guzmán Giadans
Calle 15 Guerrero y Bravo #405,
Zona Centro
Office hours: 10 am to 1 pm & 4 pm to 8 pm
Monday–Friday
Tel & Fax: (834) 3 12 74 75
E-mail: hectordiazg@hotmail.com
Universidad Autonoma de Tamaulipas,
Instituto Nacional de Ciencias de la Salud
Dr. Salvador Subiran, México, D.F.
Thirty-seven years of experience.

HOSPITALS

Centro de Salud
Centro Educativo Adolfo López Mateos
Tel: (834) 312 23 92, 312 01 36, 312 10 10

Hospital Civil 14
21 y 22 Pedro J. Mendez #502
Tel: (834) 315 05 89, 315 05 90

Hospital General de Cd. Victoria
Blvd. Fidel Velazquez #1845 Oriente,
Col. Revolución Verde
Tel: (834) 314-40 01 to 05, 316-20 17

Hospital Infantile de Tamaulipas
Calzada Luis Caballero (no street number),
Colonia Tamatan
Tel: (834) 312 93 00, 312-82 33, 312-74 62

COLIMA

DENTISTS

Dr. Juan Rafael Pinto Velasco
Calzada Galvan 137 Nte
Colonia Centro
Colima, Colima
Tel.: (312) 312-2052
Cell: (312) 317-0085

GENERAL MEDICINE

Dr. Héctor Javier Martinez Castillo
Madero 342-B
Colonia Centro
Colima, Colima
Tel.: (312) 312-8460
Cell: (312) 319-5240
Fax: (312) 330-7100

Dra. Aida Saint Martin Díaz
Constitución 564
Colonia Centro
Colima, Colima
Tel.: (312) 314-9443 /7180
Emergency: (312) 314-0769

PEDIATRICIAN

Dr. César Davila
Constitucion 564
Colonia Centro
Colima, Colima
Tel.: (312) 396-4545
Cell: (312) 320-2647

PSYCHOLOGIST

Lic. Jorge Montelongo
Moctezuma 27, Casa 3

Colonia Centro
Colima, Colima
Tel.: (312) 313-4277

PSYCHIATRIST

Dr. José Ovidio Mata Larios
Centro de Atención Médico Psiquiátrica
Maclovio Herrera 225-B
Colima, Colima
Tel.: (312) 323 5560
Cell. Emergencies: (312) 138-8758
E-mail : drjoml@yahoo.com.mx

Dr. Moisés Rozanes Tassler
Calle Gabriela Mistral 600, Depto. 4
Colima, Colima
Tel.: (312) 314-3808

HOSPITALS

Centro Médico de Colima (Private)
Maclovio Herrera 140,
Colonia Centro
Colima, Colima
Tel.: (312) 312-4044 to 46
E-mail: colimacmedico@prodigy.net.mx

Centro Hospitalario Union
Enrique Corona Morfin #90
Colonia Centro, Villa de Alvarez, Colima
Tel. (312) 311-3737

Hospital Civil Colima (Public)
Venida Elias Zamora Verduzco 1500
Colonia Arboledas
Colima, Colima
Tel.: (312) 312-0911

Hospital General Colima (Public)
San Fernando (no street number)
Colonia Lomas De Circunvalación
Colima, Colima
Tel.: (312) 313-0575

COZUMEL

CARDIOLOGISTS

Dr. Jorge Alvarez,
cell: 876-0808,
office: 872-2534

CHIROPRACTICORS

Dr. Scott Allan Kircher,
phone: 872-5099,
email: skircher28@hotmail.com

Dr. Joe Mahar,
office in Hotel Baracuda,
 phone: 872-1122

DENTISTS

Dr. Elveris,
Specialty: oral surgeon
located on 11th and 65th,
phone: 872-0808

Dr. Fernando Hernandez,
next to Farmacia Dori on Rosada Salas
 between 15 and 20,
phone: 872-0656

DIVE MEDICINE

Dr. Cardenas,
phone: 872-7087

Dr. Manuel Marin Foucher Lewis,
50 bis # 840 x 11 13 sur,
phone: 872-1616,
cell 876-0914,
email cozumeldoctor@hotmail.com

Dr. Eduardo García

General Medicine, Hyperbaric Medicine,
Diving Medicine
Address: Calle "5 Sur" #21-B
(between Avenida 5 and R.E. Melgar)
Work: (987) 872-1430
Fax: (987) 872-1848
Mobile: 044-987-111-9130
Email: dredugarcia@hotmail.com

Dr. Juan Ortegon,
phone: 872-4068

Dr. Pascual Piccolo
General Medicine, Hyperbaric Medicine
Address: Calle "6 Norte" #135 (between Ave-
nida "5 Norte" and
Avenida "10 Norte")
Work: (987) 872- 0300
Home: (987) 872-3070
Fax: (987) 872-3971
Mobile: 044-987-876-0685, 0911
Email: meditur@meditur.org

Dr. Ricardo Segovia,
phone: 872-3545, 872-5664,
872-5370, or 872-3370

EAR, NOSE & THROAT

Dr. Victor Morales
Ear, Nose & Throat, Surgery, Hyperbaric Medi-
cine, Diving Medicine
Address: Calle "1 Sur" #101
(corner of Avenida "50 Sur")
Work: (987) 872-3370
Home: (987) 872-7679
Mobile: 044-987-876-0666
Email: vicorl@hotmail.com

EMERGENCY MEDICINE

Dr. Ricardo Segovia
Emergency Medicine, General Surgery, Gastro-
enterology
Address: Calle "1 Sur" #101,
Office 1 (between Avenida "50 Sur"
and Calle "50 bis")

Work: (987) 872-9400, ext. 2210
Fax: (987) 872-9400, ext. 1011
Mobile: 044-987-876-0616
Email: ricardo.segovia@yahoo.com

GASTROENTEROLOGISTS

Dr. Ricardo Segovia
Emergency Medicine, General Surgery,
Gastroenterology
Address: Calle "1 Sur" #101,
Office 1 (between Avenida "50 Sur"
and Calle "50 bis")
Work: (987) 872-9400, ext. 2210
Fax: (987) 872-9400, ext. 1011
Mobile: 044-987-876-0616
Email: ricardo.segovia@yahoo.com

GENERAL MEDICINE

Dr. Eduardo García
General Medicine, Hyperbaric Medicine,
Diving Medicine
Address: Calle "5 Sur" #21-B
(between Avenida 5 and R.E. Melgar)
Work: (987) 872-1430
Fax: (987) 872-1848
Mobile: 044-987-111-9130
Email: dredugarcia@hotmail.com

Dr. Pascual Piccolo
General Medicine, Hyperbaric Medicine
Address: Calle "6 Norte" #135
(between Avenida "5 Norte" and
Avenida "10 Norte")
Work: (987) 872- 0300
Home: (987) 872-3070
Fax: (987) 872-3971
Mobile: 044-987-876-0685, 0911
Email: meditur@meditur.org

GYNECOLOGISTS

Dra. Guillermina Santos
Obstetrics & Gynecology
Address: Calle "1 Sur" #101

(corner of Avenida "50 Sur")
Work/Fax: 872-9400, ext. 2180
Mobile: 044-987-876-0830
Email: dragsantos@yahoo.com.mx

INTERNISTS

Dr. Eduardo Garcia Magana,
cell: 878-7988,
email: egarcia@sssnetwork.com.

Dr. Miguel Angel Ponce Duran,
cell: 101-6195

HYPERBARIC MEDICINE

Dr. Eduardo García
General Medicine, Hyperbaric Medicine,
Diving Medicine
Address: Calle "5 Sur" #21-B
(between Avenida 5 and R.E. Melgar)
Work: (987) 872-1430
Fax: (987) 872-1848
Mobile: 044-987-111-9130
Email: dredugarcia@hotmail.com

Dr. Victor Morales
Ear, Nose & Throat, Surgery, Hyperbaric Medi-
cine, Diving Medicine
Address: Calle "1 Sur" #101
(corner of Avenida "50 Sur")
Work: (987) 872-3370
Home: (987) 872-7679
Mobile: 044-987-876-0666
Email: vicorl@hotmail.com

Dr. Pascual Piccolo
General Medicine, Hyperbaric Medicine
Address: Calle "6 Norte" #135
(between Avenida "5 Norte" and
Avenida "10 Norte")
Work: (987) 872-3070
Fax: (987) 872-3971
Mobile: 044-987-876-0685
Email: meditur@meditur.org

OBSTETRICIANS

Dra. Guillermina Santos
Obstetrics & Gynecology
Address: Calle "1 Sur" #101
(corner of Avenida "50 Sur")
Work/Fax: 872-9400, ext. 2180
Mobile: 044-987-876-0830
Email: dragsantos@yahoo.com.mx

OPHTALMOLOGISTS

Dr. Concepcion Planas
San Miguel Clinic,
Tolosa-Lugo located on 10th
between Calle 1a.Sur and Avenida Juarez,
phone: 872-3805

EAR, NOSE & THROAT

Dr. Victor Morales
Ear, Nose & Throat, Surgery, Hyperbaric Medi-
cine, Diving Medicine
Address: Calle "1 Sur" #101
(corner of Avenida "50 Sur")
Work: (987) 872-3370
Home: (987) 872-7679
Mobile: 044-987-876-0666
Email: vicorl@hotmail.com

PEDIATRICIANS

Dr. Carlos García
Address: Calle "1 Sur" #101
(corner of Avenida "50 Sur")
Work/Fax: (987) 872-9400, ext. 2035
Mobile: 044-987-876-0655
Email: orcaazul55@hotmail.com

SURGEONS

Dr. Victor Morales
Ear, Nose & Throat, Surgery, Hyperbaric Medi-
cine, Diving Medicine
Address: Calle "1 Sur" #101

(corner of Avenida "50 Sur")
Work: (987) 872-3370
Home: (987) 872-7679
Mobile: 044-987-876-0666
Email: vicorl@hotmail.com

Dr. Ricardo Segovia
Emergency Medicine, General Surgery,
Gastroenterology
Address: Calle "1 Sur" #101, Office 1
(between Avenida "50 Sur" and
Calle "50 bis")
Work: (987) 872-9400, ext. 2210
Fax: (987) 872-9400, ext. 1011
Mobile: 044-987-876-0616
Email: ricardo.segovia@yahoo.com

HOSPITALS - PRIVATE

Buceo Médico Mexicano
Hyperbaric Chamber Facility
Address: Calle "5 Sur" #21-B
(between Avenida 5 and R.E. Melgar)
Borough: Colonia Centro
Main Phone #: (987) 872-1430, 1431 or 2387
Fax Phone #: (987) 872-1848
Email: cozumel@sssnetwork,
website: http://www.sssnetwork.com/mexico/
cozumel.htm

Centro Médico de Cozumel (private)
Calle 1 Sur No. 101
between 50 and 50 bis
Cozumel, Quintana Roo
Tel: (987) 872-9400 / 9401,
(987) 872-3545, 872-5664
Fax: (987) 872-3545, ext. 2007
Emergency phone: (987) 872-3545
http://costamed.com.mx/welcome/our-facilities/
cozumel-facility/
From USA Toll free 888.409.0504 ext. 1100
From inside Mexico Toll free
01800COSTAMED ext.1100
Local phone Cozumel 987.872.9400
Cell phone Cozumel 987.871.1371
Local phone Playa del Carmen 984.803.7777
Contact e-mail:

patientservices@costamed.com.mx
Supervisor e-mail:
direccion.comercial@costamed.com.mx

Clinica Villanueva
10 Av Nte x 6 # 19,
Phone: 872-0395,
doctor at home phone: 872-3050

Médica San Miguel
Calle 6 Norte No. 132
between Ave. 5 and Ave.10
Colonia Centro
Cozumel, Quintana Roo
Tel: (998) 872-0103 / 6155
Fax Phone #: (987) 872-0103, ext. 118
http://www.medicasanmiguel.com.mx/esp/index.
shtml

Médica San Miguel
Address: Calle "6 Norte" #132
(between Avenida 5 and Avenida 10)
Borough: Colonia Centro
Notable Landmarks: Near Cozumel Museum
Main Phone #: (987) 872-0103
Fax Phone #: (987) 872-0103, ext. 118

HOSPITALS - PUBLIC

Centro de Salud (Public Health Center)
11 Sur y 20 Av Sur,
872-0140 or 0525

Cruz Roja (Mexican Red Cross)
20 Av entre Rosada Salas y 1 Sur,
Phone: 872-1058,
cell phone: # 114,
public phone: 065
Treatment for donation

CUERNAVACA

CARDIOLOGISTS

Dr. Marco A. Islava
Internal Medicine, Cardiology, Interventional
Cardiology
Address: Calle Cuauhtémoc #203, Office 105
Borough: Colonia Lomas de la Selva
Work: (777) 311-2483, 313-4217
Fax: (777) 317-9366
Mobile: 044-777-328-3809
Email: docislava@msn.com, docislava@
prodigy.net.mx

FERTILITY

Dr. Gonzalo Ibinarriaga
Obstetrics & Gynecology, Fertility and Sterility
Address: Calle Cuahtemoc #203, Office 101
Borough: Colonia Lomas de la Selva
Work: (777) 313-4226
Home: (777) 102-3133
Mobile: 044-777-140-2659
Email: ibisov@hotmail.com

GYNECOLOGISTS

Dr. Gonzalo Ibinarriaga
Obstetrics & Gynecology, Fertility and Sterility
Address: Calle Cuahtemoc #203, Office 101
Borough: Colonia Lomas de la Selva
Work: (777) 313-4226
Home: (777) 102-3133
Mobile: 044-777-140-2659
Email: ibisov@hotmail.com

Dra. Dilys M. Walker
Obstetrics & Gynecology
Address: Avenida Alta Tensión #580
Borough: Colonia Cantarranas
Work: (777) 318-7563
Mobile: 044-777-327-1870

INTERNISTS

Dr. Ocampo
Av. Álvaro Obregón No. 107
Colonia Centro. CP: 62000
Cuernavaca, Morelos, México
Tel: (52)(777)3188101

Dr. Marco A. Islava
Internal Medicine, Cardiology, Interventional
Cardiology
Address: Calle Cuauhtémoc #203, Office 105
Borough: Colonia Lomas de la Selva
Work: (777) 311-2483, 313-4217
Fax: (777) 317-9366
Mobile: 044-777-328-3809
Email: docislava@msn.com,
docislava@prodigy.net.mx

OBSTETRICIAN

Dr. Gonzalo Ibinarriaga
Obstetrics & Gynecology, Fertility and Sterility
Address: Calle Cuahtemoc #203, Office 101
Borough: Colonia Lomas de la Selva
Work: (777) 313-4226
Home: (777) 102-3133
Mobile: 044-777-140-2659
Email: ibisov@hotmail.com

Dra. Dilys M. Walker
Obstetrics & Gynecology
Address: Avenida Alta Tensión #580
Borough: Colonia Cantarranas
Work: (777) 318-7563
Mobile: 044-777-327-1870

ORTHOPEDICIANS

Dr. José Luis Díaz
Orthopedics/Traumatology
Address: Calle Cuauhtémoc #203, Office 110
Borough: Colonia Lomas de la Selva
Work/Fax: (777) 317-5825
Mobile: 044-777-328-6829

PEDIATRICIAN

Dra. Rebeca Borgaro
Address: Avenida Alta Tensión #580, Office 3
Borough: Colonia Cantarranas
Work/Fax: (777) 318-7563
Mobile: 044-777-327-3623
Email: rebor@hotmail.com

TRAUMATOLOGISTS

Dr. José Luis Díaz
Orthopedics/Traumatology
Address: Calle Cuauhtémoc #203, Office 110
Borough: Colonia Lomas de la Selva
Work/Fax: (777) 317-5825
Mobile: 044-777-328-6829

HOSPITALS

Clinica Borda
Av. Álvaro Obregón No. 107
Colonia Centro. CP: 62000
Cuernavaca, Morelos, México
Telefonos: (52)(777)3188101- 3184250

Hospital Inovamed
Address: Calle Cuauhtémoc #305
(corner of Calle "5 de Mayo")
Borough: Colonia Lomas de la Selva
Notable Landmarks:
Near Hotel Suites Paraiso
Main Phone #: (777) 311-2482, 311-2483, 311-2484, 311-2485, 311-2489
Fax Phone #: (777) 311-2482, ext. 159 or 139

CULIACAN

CARDIOLOGISTS

Manuel Odin de Los Rios Ibarra
Hospital Angeles Culiacan

Blvd. Alfonso G. Calderon 2193-A Pte.
Int. 802
Desarrollo Urbano Tres Rios
Culiacan, Sinaloa,
Phone: (667) 758-7944, 758-7900 Ext. 5802
Cel: (667) 751-1662
E-Mail: odindelosrios@gmail.com
coordinacion.drodin@gmail.com

DENTISTS

Dr. Armando Aispuro Felix
Specialty: Orthodontist
Benito Juarez 390 Oriente
Colonia Centro
Culiacan, Sinaloa,
Phone: (667) 713-5457
Fax (667) 712-7890
E-Mail: aaf@ortoaispuro.com

Dr. Francisco Javier Garcia Aispuro
Specialty: Orthodontist
Benito Juarez 390 Oriente
Colonia Centro
Culiacan, Sinaloa,
Phone: (667) 713-5457
Fax (667) 712-7890
E-Mail: fga@ortoaispuro.com

Dr. Carlos Alberto San Yuriar
Specialty: General, Dental Rehabilitation
Aldama #456 Sur
Colonia Miguel Aleman
Culiacan, Sinaloa,
Phone: (667) 712-0816
E-Mail: dr_csanyuriar@hotmail.com

Dr. Juan Francisco Villalobos Guerrero
Specialty: Periodontics
Av. Alvaro Obregon #1298 Sur
Colonia Guadalupe
Culiacan, Sinaloa
Phone: (667) 716-7272
Fax: (667) 713-2464
E-Mail: endopaco@cln.megared.net.mx

EAR, NOSE, & THROAT

Dr. Ernesto Echeverria Aispuro
Hospital Angeles Culiacan
Blvd. Alfonso G. Calderon 2193-A Pte.
Int. 702 A
Desarrollo Urbano Tres Rios
Culiacan, Sinaloa,
Phone/Fax: (667) 758-7938
721-5200, 758-7900 Ext. 5702
E-Mail: drechevarria@medicosculiacan.com

Dr. Francisco Guillermo Olivera Jones,
Head & Neck Surgeon
Hospital Angeles Culiacan Blvd. Alfonso G.
Calderon 2193-A Pte. Int. 502
Desarrollo Urbano Tres Rios
Culiacan, Sinaloa
Phone: (667) 712-2872, 758-7927

ENDOCRINOLOGISTS

Dr. David Obesos Murillo
Hospital Angeles Culiacan
Blvd. Alfonso G. Calderon 2193-A Pte.
Int. 104
Desarrollo Urbano Tres Rios
Culiacan, Sinaloa
Phone: (667) 758-7904
E-Mail: dakov@pacificnet.com.mx
damdak@gmail.com

GYNECOLOGISTS/ OBSTETRICIANS

Dr. Francisco Garzon Lopez
Gynecology
(see below)

Dr. Oscar Garzon Lopez
Obstetrics
(see below)

Hospital Angeles Culiacan
Blvd. Alfonso G. Calderon 2193-A Pte.
Int. 701

Desarrollo Urbano Tres Rios
Culiacan, Sinaloa,
Phone: (667) 758-7937
Cel: (667) 107-1423
Cel: (667) 751-0621
E-Mail: dr_franciscogarzon@hotmail.com ogarzonl59@gmail.com

INTERNISTS

Dr. Ricardo Antonio Chain Castro
Hopital Angeles Culiacan
Blv. Alfonso G. Calderon 2193-A Poniente Interior 302
Desarrollo Urbano Tres Rios
Culiacan, Sinaloa,
PH: (667) 758-7914, 758-7915
E-Mail: rchaincastro21@yahoo.com.mx

Dr. Jose Tamayo
Gastroenterology
Hospital Angeles Culiacan
Blvd. Alfonso G. Calderon 2193-A Pte.
Int. 606
Desarrollo Urbano Tres Rios
Culiacan, Sinaloa,
Phone: (667) 758-7936
Cel: (667) 791-8105
E-Mail: castrotamayo@gmail.com

OPHTALMOLOGISTS

Dr. Federico V. Bazua Agerrebere
Emigdio Flores y Ponce de Leon 1248-1
Colonia Chapultepec
Culiacan, Sinaloa,
PH: (667) 713-2120, 716-7811
Fax: (667) 713-2120
E-Mail: drfbaz@colaser.com.mx

ORTHOPEDICS / TRAUMATOLOGY

Dr. Jorge Luis de La Vega,
CEMSI Policlinica Orthopedics

M. Hidalgo #251 Oriente
Colonia Centro
Culiacan, Sinaloa,
Phone: (667) 713-5281
Fax: (667) 715-7202
E-Mail: drjorgedelavega@hotmail.com

Dr. Antonio Alfredo Juan Jacobo
Orthopedics and tramatology
Obregon y Rio San Lorenzo 1106
Colonia Guadalupe
Culiacan, Sinaloa,
Tel: (667) 712-7600

PATHOLOGISTS

Dr. Agustin Ernesto Aguirre Niebla
Francisco Villa #260 Oriente
Colonia Centro, Culiacan, Sinaloa
Phone/Fax: (667) 715-3091
E-Mail: draguirreniebla@hotmail.com
cancerypatologia@hotmail.com

PEDIATRICIANS

Dr. Octavio Ruben Aguilar Bernal
Blvd. Leyva Solano #50 Ote.
Colonia Almada
Culiacan, Sinaloa,
Phone: (667) 712-1312, 716-0428, 712-0951

Dr. Marco Antonio Loaiza Arellano
Angel Flores 680 Poniente
Colonia Centro, Culiacan, Sinaloa,
Phone: (667) 7153881
E-Mail: marcoloaiza@hotmail.com

SURGEONS

Dr. Jose Ramiro Madrid Franco,
Hospital Angeles Culiacan Surgical Oncology
Blvd. Alfonso G. Calderon 2193-A Pte.
Int. 806
Desarrollo Urbano Tres Rios
Culiacan, Sinaloa,
Phone: (667) 758-7948
E-Mail: ramiromadrid@yahoo.com

Dr. Ricardo Zamudio Armenta
Francisco Villa y Corona #291 Oriente
Culiacan, Sinaloa,
Phone/Fax: (667) 713-0802
E-Mail: zam571@hotmail.com

HOSPITALS

Clinica de La Mujer
Escobedo oriente y Vicente Guerrero no. 817
Culiacan, Sinaloa,
Phone: (667) 715-3829

Cruz Roja
Blvd. Gabriel Leyva Solano 999
Culiacan, Sinaloa,
Phone: (667) 712-1994

Hospital Angeles de Culiacan
Blvd. Alfonso G. Calderon 2193 Pte.
Desarrollo Urbano Tres Rios
Culiacan, Sinaloa,
Phone: (667) 758-7700

Hospital Civil de Culiacan
Ave. Alvaro Obregon 1422 Nte. Esq.
Mariano Abasolo
Col. Tierra Blanca Culiacan, Sinaloa,
Phone: (667) 758-0500 – 715-6073

Hospital General de Culiacan
Juan Aldama (no street number)
Col. Antonio Rosales
Culiacan, Sinaloa,
Phone: (667) 712-3889 – 716-9851

Hospital Pediatrico de Sinaloa
Blvd. Constitucion 530
Col. Jorge Almada
Culiacan, Sinaloa,
Phone: 713-3523

Sanatorio Batiz Ramos
Mariano Escobedo 324 Centro
Culiacan, Sinaloa, .
Phone: (667) 712-0003

Sanatorio Cemsi Chapultepec
Blvd. Anaya 400
Col Chapultepec
Culiacan, Sinaloa
Phone (667) 715-1415

DURANGO

HOSPITALS

Hospital General de Durango
5 de Febrero y Norma Fuentes
(no street number), Zona Centro
Durango, Durango
Telephone (618) 813-0011

Hospital General de Gomez Palacio
La Salle 2 y Héroe De Nacozari
(no street number), Col. Bella Vista
Gomez Palacio, Durango
Telephone (871) 714-5522, 5858 & 5959
Fax (871) 714-7055

Hospital San Jorge
Libertad #249 Sur,
Col. Nueva Vizcaya
Durango, Durango,
Telephone (618) 817-2210

ENSENADA

CARDIOLOGISTS

Dr. Marco Antonio Susarrey
Avenida Obregón 787
Tel: (646) 178-2985
Home: (646) 178-1209
Cel: 044-646-185-0663
e-mail: cardiomed1@hotmail.com

GYNECOLOSISTS

Dr. José Luis Bastida
Calle Arenas #151. Suite 16
Borough: Playa Ensenada
Tel: (646) 176-0913
Home: (646) 177-0639
Cel: 044-646-947-7285
e-mail: docjoseluisbm@hotmail.com

INTERNISTS

Dr. Carlos Arenas Díaz
Calle Cuarta 237-2 corner with Moctezuma
Zona Centro
Ensenada, Baja California
Tel: (646) 178-3566

Dr. Armando Lievana
Calle Arenas #151
Tel: (646) 177-1340
Fax: (646) 177-2266
Cel: 044-646-171-7549
e-mail: untopo@hotmail.com

Dr. Robert Martain A.
Calle Arenas # 151, Suite 18 (3rd Floor)
Tel: (646) 177-3222
Cel: 044-646-171-7004
e-mail: rmartain@hotmail.com

Dr. Marco Antonio Susarrey
Avenida Obregón 787
Tel: (646) 178-2985
Home: (646) 178-1209
Cel: 044-646-185-0663
e-mail: cardiomed1@hotmail.com

NEPHROLOGISTS

Dr. Robert Martain A.
Calle Arenas # 151,
Suite 18 (3rd Floor)
Tel: (646) 177-3222
Cel: 044-646-171-7004
e-mail: rmartain@hotmail.com

OBSTETRICIANS

Dr. José Luis Bastida
Calle Arenas #151. Suite 16
Borough: Playa Ensenada
Tel: (646) 176-0913
Home: (646) 177-0639
Cel: 044-646-947-7285
e-mail: docjoseluisbm@hotmail.com

ORTHOPEDICS

Dr. Ricardo Garduño
Blvd. Ramírez Méndez #300
Fracc. Bahía
e-mail: r@garduno.net
176-4604
176-7495

PEDIATRICIANS

Dr. Joel Velasco
Calle Arenas #151
Borough: Playa Ensenada
Tel/Fax: (646) 173-4500
Cel: 044-646-171-5132
Email: velascoj@hospitalvelmar.com

UROLOGISTS

Dr. Alfonso Torres Badillo
Dra. Eva Chávez Vanet
Calle Cuarta 237 corner with Moctezuma
Zona Centro
Ensenada, Baja California
Tel: (646) 178-2802

HOSPITALS

Hospital Cardiomed
Avenida Obregón #1018
(between Calle 10 and 11)
Zona Centro
Notable Landmarks:
Near the Monumento a la Madre

Main/Fax Phone #: (646) 178-0351, 174-0545 (request fax tone)

Hospital Velmar
Arenas 151
Fraccionamiento Playa Ensenada
Tel/Fax #: (646) 173-4500 (request fax tone)
Website: www.hospitalvelmar.com

GUADALAJARA

GENERAL PRACTITIONERS

Dr. Gustavo Garcia Garcia
Office: Tarascos 3422
Guadalajara, Jalisco
Tel: 38130540
Cel: 044-333-579-8540

Dr. Carlos Perez Watanabe
Office: Tarascos 3422
Guadalajara, Jalisco
Tel: 3813-05-40 & 3813-05-47

CARDIOLOGISTS

Dr. Alfredo Campoy Diaz
Office: Alberta No. 1470
Guadalajara, Jalisco
Tel: 3642-14-87; 3642-5304
Cel: 044-33-1366-8831

Dr. José Adrian Carrera
Terranova 676-206
Col. Lomas Providencia
Guadalajara, Jalisco
Tel: (33) 3642-5100 / 9745
Emergencies: (33) 3678-4300 PIN# 2325

Dr. Jesús E. Esparragoza
Internal Medicine, Cardiology
Address: Calle Pablo Neruda #3265,

Office 35, 3rd Floor
Borough: Colonia Providencia
Work: (33) 3640-1104
Fax: (33) 3640-3138
Home: (33) 3641-9780
Mobile: 044-33-3677-6656
Pager: (33) 3678-4300, PIN# 18638
Email: jesparragoza@hotmail.com

Dr. Salvador E. Flores
Internal Medicine, Cardiology, Interventional Cardiology, Sports Medicine
Chapala Address: Carretera Oriente #33
Borough: Colonia Centro
Chapala Work: (376) 766-0662, 766-0500
Guadalajara Address: Tarascos #3422
Borough: Fraccionamiento Monraz
Guadalajara Work: (33) 3813-0540, 3813-0547
Home: 01-33-3641-9021
Mobile: 01-33-3105-2773
Pager: 01-33-1515-1111, PIN# 3012

Dr. Gustavo Aldofo Garcia Garcia
Office: Tarascos 3422
Guadalajara, Jalisco
Tel: 3813-0540
Cel: 044-333-579-8540

Dr. Efrain Gaxiola
Internal Medicine, Cardiology & Interventional Cardiology
Address: Calle Eulogia Parra #2969
Borough: Colonia Prados Providencia
Work: (33) 3642-0661, 3642-0651, 3641-0358
Fax: (33) 3827-1670
Mobile: 044-33-3157-6264
Pager: (33) 3678-4300, PIN# 306304
Email: efraingaxiola@yahoo.com

Dr. Sergio J. Nájar-López
Internal Medicine, Cardiology & Interventional Cardiology
Address: Avenida Hidalgo #930
Borough: Colonia Centro
Work: (33) 3825-4365, 3563-3903
Fax: (33) 3827-1670

Mobile: 044-33-3676-1625,
044-333-954-2645
Pager: (33) 3678-4300, PIN# 9500062
Email: sergionajar@yahoo.com

Dr. Michael C. Ritota Jr.
Internal Medicine, Cardiology
Address: Calle Tarascos #3422
Borough: Fraccionamiento Monraz
Work: (33) 3813-0547, 3813-0554,
3813-0540
Fax: (33) 3813-0857
Home: (33) 3641-0338
Mobile: 044-33-3676-2714
Email: mikeritota@mexis.com

Dr. Victor Orendain
Tarascos 3469 - 1st floor
Col. Monraz
Guadalajara, Jalisco
Tel: (33) 3813-3003 / 3004
Emergencies: (33) 3678-4300 PIN# 18505

CARDIOVASCULAR SURGEONS

Dr. Gustavo A. Rubio Arguello
Office: Av. Empresarios 150
15th floor, Torre Elite
Guadalajara, Jalisco
Tel: 3813-30-10, 3848-55-05
Cel: 044-333-667-8077

DERMATOLOGISTS

Dra. Norma Gabriela Campos Cornejo
Office: Garibaldi 2561
Guadalajara, Jalisco
Tel: 3630-22-18
Cel: 044-333-662-9441

Dra. Angelina Gonzalez Rios
Office: Tarascos 3432
Guadalajara, Jalisco
Tel: 3813-31-54 / 3813-20-05 /
3813-21-61

DENTISTS

Dr. Carlos A. Rodriguez
Office: Angulo 2517
Guadalajara, Jalisco
Tel: 3615-8802

EAR, NOSE & THROAT

Dr. Rigoberto Astorga del Toro
Office:Tarascos 3473
6to piso consultorio 630-A
Tel: 3648-34-29 / 3648-34-31

Dr. Carlos Marin Camarena
Office: Tarascos 3469 - 510
Tel: 3813-30-18
Cel: 044-333-100-6257

Dr. Carlos M. Radillo Martinez Sandoval
Office: Vallarta 3012
Guadalajara, Jalisco
Tel: 3616-38-82

GASTROENTEROLOGISTS

Dr. Bernardo Lancaster Jones
Office: Tarascos 3432 -14
Guadalajara, Jal.
Tel: 3813-2090
Cel: 044-333-100-3317

Dr. Antonio Orozco
Office: Jose Maria Robles 792
Colonia Chapalita
Guadalajara, Jalisco
Tel: 3647-56-00 &
3647-72-51
Nextel: 3944-4339

Dr. Fernado Pérez Barba
Office: Tarascos 3422
Guadalajara, Jalisco
Tel: 3813-0540
Cel: 044-333-156-3174

Dr. Jaime Ramirez Parra, F.A.C.P.
Office: Tarascos 3514

Tel: 3120-46-55 / 3120-46-82
Cel: 044-333-807-5662

Dr. Pablo J. Robles
General Surgery, Laparoscopic & Endoscopic
Gastroenterology
Address: Calle Tarascos #3432
Borough: Fraccionamiento Monraz
Work/Fax: (33) 3813-2090
Home: (33) 3641-9982
Mobile: 044-33-3100-2097
Pager: (33) 3669-0579, PIN# 5252521
Email: pablojroblesp@hotmail.com

GERIATRICS

Dr. Victor Fernando Villa Esteves
Office: Terranova 676 - 205
Guadalajara, Jalisco
Tel: 3641-78-10 & 3641-78-03
Cel: 044-331-090-0991

Dr. Leonardo Fernandez Cruz
Office: Luis Perez Verdia No.260
Guadalajara, Jalisco
Tel: 3615-2561
Cel: 044-33-357-66713

GYNECOLOGISTS

Dr. Carlos R. Villareal
Obstetrics & Gynecology, Laparoscopy
Address: Calle Tarascos #3514,
Office 7
Borough: Fraccionamiento Monraz
Work: (33) 3813-0440, 3120-4655
Fax: (33) 3344-5140
Pager: (33) 3678-4300, PIN# 18161
Email: cvillarrealclauss@hotmail.com

INTERNISTS

Dr. Fernando de la Cueva
Office: Av. Nino Obrero 1097 - 102
Tel: 3122-10-69 & 3122-09-53
Cel: 044-333-105-9579

Dr. Carlos Dueñas
Address: Calle Pablo Casals #657,
Office 302
Borough: Colonia Prados Providencia
Work: (33) 3669-0222, ext 3111
Fax: (33) 3642-0754
Home: (33) 3642-0754
Mobile: 044-33-3677-9207
Pager: (33) 3630-3131, PIN# 40031
Email: dirmed@sanjavier.com.mx

Dr. Jesús E. Esparragoza
Internal Medicine, Cardiology
Address: Calle Pablo Neruda #3265,
Office 35, 3rd Floor
Borough: Colonia Providencia
Work: (33) 3640-1104
Fax: (33) 3640-3138
Home: (33) 3641-9780
Mobile: 044-33-3677-6656
Pager: (33) 3678-4300, PIN# 18638
Email: jesparragoza@hotmail.com

Dr. Carlos Fadl Adib
Office: Puerta de Hierro 5150
Torre A, 6th floor # 604
Tel: 1368-2064 & 3640-2000
Cel: 044-333-662-9294

Dr. Fernando de la Cueva
Office: Av. Nino Obrero 1097 - 102
Tel: 3122-10-69 & 3122-09-53
Cel: 044-333-105-9579

Dr. Salvador E. Flores
Internal Medicine, Cardiology, Interventional
Cardiology, Sports Medicine
Chapala Address: Carretera Oriente #33
Borough: Colonia Centro
Chapala Work: (376) 766-0662, 766-0500
Guadalajara Address: Tarascos #3422
Borough: Fraccionamiento Monraz
Guadalajara Work: (33) 3813-0540,
3813-0547
Home: 01-33-3641-9021
Mobile: 01-33-3105-2773
Pager: 01-33-1515-1111, PIN# 3012

Dr. Efrain Gaxiola
Internal Medicine, Cardiology & Interventional
Cardiology
Address: Calle Eulogia Parra #2969
Borough: Colonia Prados Providencia
Work: (33) 3642-0661, 3642-0651,
3641-0358
Fax: (33) 3827-1670
Mobile: 044-33-3157-6264
Pager: (33) 3678-4300, PIN# 306304
Email: efraingaxiola@yahoo.com

Dra. Berenice Lopez
Tarascos 3469-3rd floor
Guadalajara, Jalisco
Tel: (33) 3813-2945
Emergencies: (33) 3678-4300 PIN# 324

Dr. Eloy Medina
Address: Planta Alta Tarascos #3473,
Office 540A
Borough: Fraccionamiento Monraz
Work: (33) 3813-0042, Ext. 5510
Fax: (33) 3344-5140
Mobile: 044-33-3676-0310
Pager: (33) 1515-1111, PIN# 3513

Dr. Sergio J. Nájar-López
Internal Medicine, Cardiology & Interventional
Cardiology
Address: Avenida Hidalgo #930
Borough: Colonia Centro
Work: (33) 3825-4365, 3563-3903
Fax: (33) 3827-1670
Mobile: 044-33-3676-1625
Pager: (33) 3678-4300, PIN# 9500062
Email: sergionajar@yahoo.com

Dr. Michael C. Ritota Jr.
Internal Medicine, Cardiology
Address: Calle Tarascos #3422
Borough: Fraccionamiento Monraz
Work: (33) 3813-0547, 3813-0554,
3813-0540
Fax: (33) 3813-0857
Home: (33) 3641-0338
Mobile: 044-33-3676-2714
Email: mikeritota@mexis.com

LAPAROSCOPY

Dr. Carlos R. Villareal
Obstetrics & Gynecology, Laparoscopy
Address: Calle Tarascos #3514, Office 7
Borough: Fraccionamiento Monraz
Work: (33) 3813-0440, 3120-4655
Fax: (33) 3344-5140
Pager: (33) 3678-4300, PIN# 18161
Email: cvillarrealclauss@hotmail.com

NEPHROLOGISTS

Dr. Juan Fernandez de Castro
Office: Tarascos 3469 - 307
Guadalajara, Jalisco
Tel: 3813-32-52
Cel: 33-13088870

Dr. Gilberto Hernandez Alvarez
Office: Av. Americas 137
Guadalajara, Jalisco
Tel: 3615-98-23 & 3615-39-69
Cel: 044-3137-1489

NEUROLOGIST

Dr. Alfredo Cornejo Aguiar
Office: Empresarios 150
Tarascos 3473 Office # 340
Torre Elite, Puerta de Hierro
Tel: 3640-00-69
Cel: 0443-661-4561

OBSTETRICS/
GYNECOLOGY

Dr. Luis Gerardo Orozco Ibarra
Office: Homero 200, Fracc. Monraz
Guadalajara, Jalisco
Tel: 3813-3230 & 3813-3229

Dr. Marco Antonio Rodríguez Rosales
Unidad Médica San Lucas
Tarasco #3213
Guadalajara, Jalisco

Tel: 3813-2061 / 3813-2032

Dr. Carlos R. Villareal
Obstetrics & Gynecology, Laparoscopy
Address: Calle Tarascos #3514, Office 7
Borough: Fraccionamiento Monraz
Work: (33) 3813-0440, 3120-4655
Fax: (33) 3344-5140
Pager: (33) 3678-4300, PIN# 18161
Email: cvillarrealclauss@hotmail.com

ONCOLOGISTS

Dr. Horacio Alatorre /
Dr. Jorge Jimenez /
Dr. Gilberto Morgan /
Dr. Juan A. Olguin
Office: Juan Palomar y Arias 530
Guadalajara, Jalisco
Tel: 3641-5081 & 3642-9509
Cel: 044-333-809-4365 /
044-333-809-4554

OPHTALMOLOGISTS

Dr. Ricardo Cruz Perez
Office: Pedro Moreno 1103
Guadalajara, Jalisco
Tel: 3825-30-15 & 3825-97-24
Cel: 044-333-189-5928

Dr. Rene Santillan Lomas
Office: Tarascos 3469 - 215
Guadalajara, Jalisco
Tel: 3813-11-74 / 3642-72-53

ORTHOPEDICS / TRAUMATOLOGY

Dr. Jose Carrillo Perez
Office: Manuel Acuna 3310
Guadalajara, Jalisco
Tel: 3642-9985
Fax: 3640-2780
Cel: 044-333-148-3225

Dr. Juan Ramon Cisneros Ochoa
Office: Av. La Paz 2758
Col. Arcos Sur
Guadalajara, Jalisco
Tel: 3630-1355

Dr. Ramiro Flores Moreno
Office: Av. Nino Obrero 850
Guadalajara, Jalisco
Tel: 3647-6684
Nextel: 1484-2453

Dr. Guillmero Navarro Gomez
Piso 2º Suite #213
Guadalajara, Jalisco
Tel: 3813-3063
Cel: 044-333-359-9460

Dr. Jose Palomar Lever
Office: Av. Union 163, 3rd floor
Tel:3616-00-48
Cel: 044-333-100-2165

PEDIATRICIANS

Dra. Dalia Aleman Robleto
Office: Pablo Neruda 3265
Guadalajara, Jalisco
Tel: 3640-0295 & 3641-6720

Dr. Sergio Alejandro Estrada A.
Office: Eulogio Parra 2969
Guadalajara, Jalisco
Tel: 3642-3648
Cel: 044-333-895-6305

Dr. Roberto Martínez-Carboney
Pediatrics
Address: Calle Pablo Casals #640
Borough: Colonia Prados Providencia
Work: (33) 3669-0222, ext. 3075
Fax: (33) 3669-0222
Home: (33) 3632-6039
Mobile: 044-33-3288-3180
Pager: (33) 1515-1111, PIN# 3490
Email: carboney@sanjavier.com.mx

Dr. Eduardo J. Velasco-Sánchez

Pediatrics
Address: Avenida Aztecas #280,
Office 1 (between Toltecas and Mayas)
Borough: Fraccionamiento Monraz
Work/Fax: (33) 3641-6015
Mobile: 044-33-3809-2346
Pager: (33) 3630-3131, PIN#: 40014
Email: eduardovelasco@megared.net.mx

PLASTIC SURGEONS

Dr. Manuel Jimenez del Torro
Office: Tarascos 3514
Guadalajara, Jalisco
Tel: 3813-0700
Cel: 044-333-106-5980

PROCTOLOGISTS

Dr. Victor M. Maciel Gutierrez
Office: Jose Maria Heredia 2980
Guadalajara, Jalisco
Tel: 3641-4305

PSYCHATRISTS

Dr. Pedro Pablo Alvarez
Office: Eulogio Parra #3061
Guadalajara, Jalisco
Tel: 3641-8043 / 3642-5146 / 3641-4262

Dr. Alvaro Zomoza Matthews
Office: Justo Sierra 2310
Guadalajara, Jalisco
Tel: 3616-4492 & 3616-1089
Cel: 333-6629724

RHEUMATOLOGISTS

Dr. Javier Orozco-Alcala
Office: Reforma 2491
Guadalajara, Jalisco
Tel: 3616-1680
Fax: 3616-2840

SPORTS MEDICINE

Dr. Salvador E. Flores
Internal Medicine, Cardiology, Interventional
Cardiology, Sports Medicine
Chapala Address: Carretera Oriente #33
Borough: Colonia Centro
Chapala Work: (376) 766-0662, 766-0500
Guadalajara Address: Tarascos #3422
Borough: Fraccionamiento Monraz
Guadalajara Work: (33) 3813-0540,
3813-0547
Home: 01-33-3641-9021
Mobile: 01-33-3105-2773
Pager: 01-33-1515-1111, PIN# 3012

SURGEONS

Dr. Narcizo León
General Surgery
Address: Calle Pablo Casals #657,
Office 103
Borough: Colonia Prados Providencia
Work: (33) 3642-6623
Fax: (33) 3642-2195
Pager: (33) 3678-4300, PIN# 18607
Mobile: 044-33-3667-7030
Email: narcizoleon@msn.com

Dr. Pablo J. Robles
General Surgery, Laparoscopic & Endoscopic
Gastroenterology
Address: Calle Tarascos #3432
Borough: Fraccionamiento Monraz
Work/Fax: (33) 3813-2090
Home: (33) 3641-9982
Mobile: 044-33-3100-2097
Pager: (33) 3669-0579, PIN# 5252521
Email: pablojroblesp@hotmail.com

UROLOGISTS

Dr. Daniel Vázquez Pérez
Office: Tarascos 3422
Guadalajara, Jalisco
Tel: 3813-0540
Cel: 044-333-105-0603

HOSPITALS

Hospital Americas (Sharp)
Av. Americas 932
Sector Hidalgo
Guadalajara, Jalisco
Tel: (33) 3817-3141 / 0478
Fax: (33) 3817-3004

Hospital Angeles del Carmen
Address: Calle Tarascos #3435 (at the corner of
Calle Lacandones)
Borough: Fraccionamiento/Colonia Monraz
Notable Landmarks: Behind Plaza México
Main Phone #: (33) 3813-0042
Fax Phone #: (33) 3813-3463
Emergency Phone #: (33) 3813-1224
Website: www.mediks.com

Hospital Arboledas Av. Nicolas Copernico 4000
Guadalajara, Jalisco
Tel. 3631-3051 / 3631-4450

Hospital Bernadette
Address: Avenida Hidalgo #930 (1½ blocks
from Calle Enrique Díaz de León)
Borough: Colonia Centro
Notable Landmarks: Downtown area
Main Phone #: (33) 3825-4365
Fax Phone #: (33) 3826-8585

Hospital Civil de Guadalajara
Hospital 278
Col. El Retiro
Guadalajara, Jalisco
Tel: (33) 3614-5501 / 7531
Fax: (33) 3614-7711

Hospital Del Carmen
Tarascos 3435
Col. Monraz
Guadalajara, Jalisco
Tel: (33) 3813-0042 / 0078
Fax: (33) 3813-0042 ext.255

Hospital México Americano
Colomos 2110
Col. Ladron de Guevara

Guadalajara, Jalisco
Tel and Fax: (33) 3648-3333/4

Hospital San Javier
Address: Avenida Pablo Casals #640
Borough: Colonia Prados Providencia
Notable Landmarks:
Two blocks from Manuel Acuña Avenue
Main Phone #: (33) 3669-0222
Fax Phone #: (33) 3669-0222, ext. 3110
Emergency Phone #: (33) 3641-4832
www.sanjavier.com.mx

Hospital Santa Margarita
Garibaldi 880
Guadalajara, Jalisco
Tel: 3825-33-05 / 3826-5630; 3825-3072

Nuevo Hospital Civil de Guadalajara
(Specialties)
Salvador Quevedo y Zubieta 750
Col. El Retiro
Guadalajara City, Jalisco
Tel: (33) 3618-0077
Fax: (33) 3618-0024

Sanatorio Guadalajara Justo
Sierra 2130
Guadalajara, Jalisco
Tel: 3616-0563 / 3616-8768 / 3615-0379

Sanatorio San Francisco de Asis
Av. Américas 1946
Guadalajara, Jalisco
Tel: 3817-5017 / 3817-5034 / 3817-5020

GUANAJUATO

GENERAL MEDICINE

Dr. Alberto G. Mora
General Medicine, Intensive Care
Address: Calle Paseo de la Prensa #85
Borough: Colonia Centro

Work/Fax: (473) 731-1070
Home: (473) 733-1213
Mobile: 044-473-103-0113
Email: dr_alberto1145@hotmail.com

INTENSIVE CARE

Dr. Alberto G. Mora
General Medicine, Intensive Care
Address: Calle Paseo de la Prensa #85
Borough: Colonia Centro
Work/Fax: (473) 731-1070
Home: (473) 733-1213
Mobile: 044-473-103-0113
Email: dr_alberto1145@hotmail.com

INTERNISTS

Dr. Jesús A. Sánchez
Internal Medicine
Address: Plaza de la Paz #20
Work/Fax: (473) 732-0005
Mobile: 044-473-738-0229
Email: dradolfolevya@hotmail.com,
drsleyva@prodigy.net.mx

HOSPITALS

Médica Integral Guanajuatense
Address: Plaza de la Paz # 20
Borough: Zona Centro
Notable Landmarks:
Near Basílica and Tourist Center
Main Phone #: (473) 732-2305
Fax Phone #: (473) 732-6985

GUAYMAS

GENERAL MEDICINE

Dr. Gregorio V. Sánchez
General Medicine
Address: Avenida Gregorio Sánchez
Márquez #32 (between Calle 19 and
Calle 20)
Town: Guaymas
Work: (662) 222-0766
Fax: (662) 222-0267
Mobile: 044-662-106-0645
Email: sanatoriogasanchez@hotmail.com

INTERNISTS

Dr. Reynaldo Alberto Ocampo Rivera
Serdan 690-Bis int. 1-C
Colonia Centro
Guaymas, Sonora
Tel: (622) 222-1863
Home: (622) 222-2838
E-Mail: rocampo@mail.medinet.net.mx

PEDIATRICIANS

Dr. Rubén Alberto Palestino Prudente
Ave. Serdán 690-4
Pasaje Rigollot
Guaymas, Sonora
Tel. & Fax: (662) 222-8960
Cell: (622) 228-0840
E-Mail: pales510@prodigy.net.mx
drpalestino@hotmail.com

RADIOLOGISTS

Dr. Jesus Alberto Celaya Castro
Alfonso Iberri #223 General Medicine
Guaymas, Sonora

Phone: (622) 222-1070 office,
(622) 222-3033 home
Email: jesuscelayacastro@hotmail.com

HOSPITALS

Hospital General de Guaymas (Semeson)
Calle 15 entre Avenidas 7 y 8
Colonia Centro
Guaymas, Sonora,
Phone/fax: (622) 224-0138

Pabellon Guadalupe
Ave. 6 y Calle 11
Guaymas, Sonora
Tel: (622) 222-0485 222-4009,
Fax: 224-3350
Email: dadivitanac@hotmail.com

Sanatorío G. A. Sanchez
Avenida 15 No. 32
Colonia Centro
Guaymas, Sonora
Tel: (622) 222-0766 / 0267
Email: sanatoriogasanchez@hotmail.com

HERMOSILLO

CARDIOLOGISTS

Dr. Jesus Manuel Canale
Centro Médico del Río Internal Medicine
Reforma Sur #273
(across street from Torre Cima)
Hermosillo, Sonora
Tel: (662) 212-1857,
Fax: (662) 212-1890
email: jcanale@infosel.net.mx

Dr. Jorge Cortés
Internal Medicine, Cardiology, Clinical &
Interventional Cardiology
Address: Paseo Río San Miguel #49,

Office 406, 4th Floor, Sector "A"
Borough: Proyecto Río Sonora
Work: (662) 259-0965
Fax: (662) 259-0967
Mobile: 044-662-276-0115
Email: jcorteslaurenz@yahoo.com
Office hours: M–F: 11am–1pm, 5pm–8pm

Dr. Cesar Manuel Gudino Aguilar
Torre Cima
Paseo Rio San Miguel y Reforma
Hermosillo, Sonora,
Phone: (662) 259-9309, (662) 259-9310
Email: ceguag@yahoo.com

Dr. Rodolfo E. Siordia
Internal Medicine, Cardiology,
Cardiothoracic Surgery
Address: Paseo Río San Miguel #49,
Office #510, 4th Floor, Sector "B"
Borough: Proyecto Río Sonora
Work/Fax: (662) 259-0965
Mobile: 044-662 276-0379
Email: resiordia@yahoo.com

Dr. Arturo Siordia Zamorano
Hospital Cima
Paseo Río San Miguel No. 35
Hermosillo, Sonora
Phone: (662) 259-9323, (662) 259-9324
-Nogales office
Tel. & Fax: (631) 312-2810
E-mail: siodia@dakotacoom.net

DENTISTS

Dr. Romero Moreno Matiella
Olivares No. 142
Colonia Valle Grande
Hermosillo, Sonora
Tel: (662) 218-7790
Fax: (662) 216-6505
Email: dr.romeomoreno@gmail.com

ENDOCRINOLOGISTS

Dr. Juan A. González-Estrella
Obstetrics & Gynecology, Reproductive
Endocrinology & Sterility
Address: Paseo Río San Miguel #46,
Offices 302 & 303
Borough: Villa de Serís
Work: (662) 217-2030, 259-9313, 259-9314
Fax: (662) 217-2030
Pager: (662) 259-0333, PIN# 951
Email: dr.gonzalezestrella@hotmail.com

GASTROENTEROLOGISTS

Dr. Luis E. Enríquez
Internal Medicine, Gastroenterology
Address: Paseo Río San Miguel #49,
Office 416, 4th Floor, Sector "C"
Borough: Proyecto Río Sonora
Work: (662) 259-0959
Fax: (662) 259-0955
Home: (662) 216-9719
Mobile: 044-662-256-7036
Pager: (662) 259-2626, PIN# 5319065
Email: leemcima@hotmail.com

GYNECOLOGISTS

Dr. Juan A. González-Estrella
Obstetrics & Gynecology, Reproductive
Endocrinology & Sterility
Address: Paseo Río San Miguel #46,
Offices 302 & 303
Borough: Villa de Serís
Work: (662) 217-2030, 259-9313, 259-9314
Fax: (662) 217-2030
Pager: (662) 259-0333, PIN# 951
Email: dr.gonzalezestrella@hotmail.com

Dra. Ruth E. González-Rivera
Obstetrics & Gynecology
Address: Paseo Río San Miguel #49,
Offices 110 & 111, 1st Floor,
Sector "B"
Borough: Proyecto Río Sonora

Work: (662) 259-0950
Fax: (662) 259-0949
Mobile: 044-662-276-4631
Pager: (662) 259-0333, PIN# 1158
Email: draruth7@hotmail.com

Dr. José Maria Mojarra Estrada
Torre Médica
Paseo Río San Miguel No. 35-115
Hermosillo, Sonora
Tel: (662) 259-0959 / 0956
Fax: (662) 259-0955
E-Mail: jmojarra@rtn.uson.mx

INTERNISTS

Dr. Jorge Cortés
Internal Medicine, Cardiology, Clinical &
Interventional Cardiology
Address: Paseo Río San Miguel #49,
Office 406, 4th Floor, Sector "A"
Borough: Proyecto Río Sonora
Work: (662) 259-0965
Fax: (662) 259-0967
Mobile: 044-662-276-0115
Email: jcorteslaurenz@yahoo.com
Office hours: M–F: 11am–1pm, 5pm–8pm

Dr. Luis E. Enríquez
Internal Medicine, Gastroenterology
Address: Paseo Río San Miguel #49,
Office 416, 4th Floor, Sector "C"
Borough: Proyecto Río Sonora
Work: (662) 259-0959
Fax: (662) 259-0955
Home: (662) 216-9719
Mobile: 044-662-256-7036
Pager: (662) 259-2626, PIN# 5319065
Email: leemcima@hotmail.com

Dr. Angel Sánchez-Hudson
Internal Medicine, Diabetes
Address: Paseo Río San Miguel #49,
Office 222, 2nd Floor, Sector "C"
Borough: Proyecto Río Sonora
Work: (662) 259-0959
Fax: (662) 259-0955

Pager: (662) 259-0333, PIN# 175
Email: asanchez@cimahermosillo.com

Dr. Rodolfo E. Siordia
Internal Medicine, Cardiology,
Cardiothoracic Surgery
Address: Paseo Río San Miguel #49,
Office #510, 4th Floor, Sector "B"
Borough: Proyecto Río Sonora
Work/Fax: (662) 259-0965
Mobile: 044-662-276-0379
Email: resiordia@yahoo.com

OBSTETRICIAN

Dr. Juan A. González-Estrella
Obstetrics & Gynecology, Reproductive
Endocrinology & Sterility
Address: Paseo Río San Miguel #46,
Offices 302 & 303
Borough: Villa de Serís
Work: (662) 217-2030, 259-9313, 259-9314
Fax: (662) 217-2030
Pager: (662) 259-0333, PIN# 951
Email: dr.gonzalezestrella@hotmail.com

Dr. José Maria Mojarra Estrada
Torre Médica
Paseo Río San Miguel No. 35-115
Hermosillo, Sonora
Tel: (662) 259-0959 / 0956
Fax: (662) 259-0955
E-Mail: jmojarra@rtn.uson.mx

Dra. Ruth E. González-Rivera
Obstetrics & Gynecology
Address: Paseo Río San Miguel #49,
Offices 110 & 111, 1st Floor,
Sector "B"
Borough: Proyecto Río Sonora
Work: (662) 259-0950
Fax: (662) 259-0949
Mobile: 044-662-276-4631
Pager: (662) 259-0333, PIN# 1158
Email: draruth7@hotmail.com

ORTHOPEDICS

Dr. Jose Arturo Olivas Robles Linares
Orthopedics and Traumatology
Av. Juarez y Luis Donaldo Colosio
Hermosillo, Sonora,
Phone: (662) 213-6251,
Fax: (662) 212-1890
Torre CIMA Phone: (662) 259-9300
E-Mail: arturoolivas@hotmail.com

PATHOLOGISTS

Dr. Roberto de Leon Caballero,
Centro de Patologia Avanzada de Sonora
Juarez #118-2
Hermosillo, Sonora,
Phone/Fax: (662) 217-2439
Email: cdpas.cpa@prodigy.net.mx

PLASTIC SURGEONS

Dr. Francisco Jesus Marcos Souffle Villa Juarez
#120 Norte Surgery
Hermosillo, Sonora
Phone: (662) 214-8188,
Fax: (662) 214-6609
Cel.(044 662) 256-6319
E-Mail: soufflé_cirujano@prodigy.net.mx

Dr. Gilberto Ungson
Obesity Surgery
Address: Paseo Río San Miguel #35
Borough: Proyecto Río Sonora
Work: (662) 259-0965
Fax: (662) 259-0967
Mobile: 044-662-256-2357
Pager: (662) 259-0333, PIN# 331
Email: gungson@hotmail.com

SURGEON

Dr. Gilberto Ungson
Laparoscopic Surgery, Obesity Surgery
Address: Paseo Río San Miguel #35
Borough: Proyecto Río Sonora

Work: (662) 259-0965
Fax: (662) 259-0967
Mobile: 044-662-256-2357
Pager: (662) 259-0333, PIN# 331
Email: gungson@hotmail.com

UROLOGISTS

Dr. Alberto E. Estrada
Address: Paseo Río San Miguel #49,
Office 211, 2nd Floor, Sector "B"
Borough: Proyecto Río Sonora
Work: (662) 259-0909, 213-2000
Fax: (662) 259-0909
Mobile: 044-662-111-1215,
044-662-213-7585
Pager: (662) 259-0333, PIN# 155
Email: drestradatapia@yahoo.com.mx

HOSPITALS

Hospital Cima
Paseo Rio San Miguel #35
Hermosillo, Sonora.
Phone: (662) 251-6776,
Cell: (662) 144 1477,
Cell: (622) 196-0711,
Cell: (622) 138-0338

Centro Medico del Noroeste
Ave. Luis Donaldo Colosio 23 Ote.
Hermosillo, Sonora
Tel: (662) 217-4521
Phone: (662) 108-0900
www.clinicadelnoroeste.com

Hospital CIMA
Address: Paseo Río San Miguel #35
(between Reforma and Comonfort streets)
Borough: Proyecto Río Sonora
Notable Landmarks: Downtown, near
government buildings
Main Phone #: (662) 259-0900
Fax Phone #: (662) 259-0999
Emergency Phone #: (662) 259-0911
www.cimahermosillo.com

Toll free: 01-800-234-2462

Hospital General del Estado
Blvd. Luis Encinas
Hermosillo, Sonora
Phone: (662) 259-2500, (662) 259-2501

Hospital Infantil DIF (Children's Hosptial)
Reforma 355 Norte
Hermosillo, Sonora
Phone: (662) 289-0600

Hospital Licona
Luis Donaldo Colosio #42
on the corner of Jesus Garcia
Hermosillo, Sonora
Phone: (662) 108-4450,
Fax 213-6616
E-Mail: slicona@prodigy.net.mx
www.hospitallicona.com.mx

Hospital San Jose
Blvd. Morelos #340
Hermosillo, Sonora
Phone: (662) 109-0500
www.grupomedicosanjose.com.mx

HUATULCO

HOSPITALS

Central Medica Huatulco (Private)
Framboyant 205
La Crucecita
Bahías de Huatulco, Oaxaca
Tel: (958) 587-0104
Fax: (958) 587-0743
Emergency: (958) 587-6550

Clinica Medica Quirurgica (Private)
Dr. Ricardo Carrillo Barragan
Sabali 403, 2nd floor
Corner with Gardenia
La Crucecita

Bahías de Huatulco, Oaxaca
Tel & Fax: (958) 587-0600 / 0687
Emergency: (958) 587-6055

Cruz Roja (Public)
Blvd. Chahué 110
Bahías de Huatulco, Oaxaca
Tel: (958) 587-1188

Sanatorío Naval Militar (Public)
Bvld. Chahue, Lotes 56 y 57,
Sector "R"
La Crucecita
Bahías de Huatulco, Oaxaca
Emergencies: (958) 587-1188
Administration: (958) 587-1548 / 1118 / 1116

HUIXQUILUCAN

SURGEONS

Dr. Tomás Barrientos
Hospital Ángeles de las Lomas
Vialidad de la Barranca (no street number), Office 515
Col. Valle de las Palmas
Huixquilucan, Estado de México
Tel: (55) 5246-9566 / 69

ISLA MUJERES

GYNECOLOGISTS

Dr. Antonio Coronado-Rojas
Address: Calle Francisco I. Madero #16,
Office 1 (corner of Calle Guerrero)
Borough: Colonia Centro
Work: (998) 877-0117
Home: (998) 877-1687

OBSTETRICIAN

Dr. Antonio Coronado-Rojas
Obstetrics & Gynecology
Address: Calle Francisco I. Madero #16,
Office 1 (corner of Calle Guerrero)
Borough: Colonia Centro
Work: (998) 877-0117
Home: (998) 877-1687

SURGEONS

Dr. Demetrio Celaya
General Surgery
Address: Calle Francisco I. Madero #16,
Office 1 (corner of Calle Guerrero)
Borough: Colonia Centro
Work: (998) 877-0117
Mobile: 044-984-100-9306
Email: mayetsie@hotmail.com

IXTAPA

Hospital Naval
Ave. Paseo del Palmar (no street number)
Ixtapa, Guerrero
Tel.: (755) 553-0499 / 553-0553

IXTLAHUACAN

HOSPITAL

Hospital General Ixtlahuacan (Public)
Unidad Psiquiatrica
Zaragoza (no street number)
Ixtlahuacán, Colima
Tel: (313) 324-9045 / 9156
(only spanish spoken)

LA PAZ

HOSPITALS

Centro Médico de Diagnóstico Integral
Ave. 5 de Mayo, entre Ramírez y Altamirano
La Paz, Baja California Sur
Tel: (612) 122-3990 / 125-2200 / 123-5796

Cruz Roja
Av. de los Deportistas y Luis Donaldo Colosio
Colonia Donceles 28
La Paz, Baja California Sur
Tel: (612) 122-1111
Fax: (612) 122-1222
(Services available in Spanish only)

Unidad Médica (Military Hospital)
16 de Septiembre 1420
La Paz, Baja California Sur
Tel: (612) 122-7028 / 4417

LAZARO CARDENAS

HOSPITALS

Cruz Roja
Aldama (no street number)
Col. Centro
Lázaro Cárdenas, Michoacán
Tel: (753) 532-0575

Hospital General
Ave. Lázaro Cárdenas (no street number)
Col. Centro
Lázaro Cárdenas, Michoacán
Tel: (753) 532-0823
Emergencies: (753) 532-0822

Hospital Naval
Calle P. de la Solidaridad (no street number)
Col. Solidaridad
Lázaro Cárdenas, Michoacán
Tel: (753) 531-3611

Morelia Medica Center
Tanganxoan 89
Col. Ampliación Jarene
Lázaro Cárdenas, Michoacán
Tel: (753) 532-3687 / 537-1603
Service 24 hours
Website: http://moreliamedicacenter.com

LEON

CARDIOLOGISTS

Dr. Carlos Harrison
Internal Medicine, Cardiology, Critical Care
Address: Avenida Cerro Gordo #311,
Office 910
Borough: Colonia Fracción del Cerro Gordo
Work/Fax: (477) 788-5691
Mobile: 044-477-638-5954
Pager: 01-800-500-1212, PIN #4776385954
Email: charrison@angelesleon.com

CRITICAL CARE

Dr. Carlos Harrison
Internal Medicine, Cardiology, Critical Care
Address: Avenida Cerro Gordo #311,
Office 910
Borough: Colonia Fracción del Cerro Gordo
Work/Fax: (477) 788-5691
Mobile: 044-477-638-5954
Pager: 01-800-500-1212, PIN #4776385954
Email: charrison@angelesleon.com

GASTROENTEROLOGISTS

Dr. Ernesto Marín
General Surgery, Gastroenterology
Address: Avenida Cerro Gordo #311,
Office 610
Borough: Colonia Fracción del Cerro Gordo
Work: (477) 788-5661
Home: (477) 781-0669
Mobile: 044-477-729-1343
Email: emarin@angelesleon.com

GYNECOLOGY

Dr. Héctor López-Frisbie
Obstetrics & Gynecology
Address: Avenida Cerro Gordo #311,
Office 210
Borough: Colonia Fracción del Cerro Gordo
Work: (477) 788-5621, 788-5721
Home: (477) 781-1668
Mobile: 044-477-159-3333
Nextel: 177413*1
Email: drlopezfrisbie@gmail.com

Dra. Sara Gutiérrez
Obstetrics & Gynecology, Gynecologic
Urology
Address: Plaza de las Américas #115
Borough: Colonia Jardines del Moral
Work/Fax: (477) 714-2139, 779-0608
Pager: (477) 714-8022, PIN# 700496
Email: sgtct@hotmail.com

HEMATOLOGISTS

Dr. Carlos Ramírez-Mateos
Internal Medicine, Hematology, Immunology
Address: Avenida Cerro Gordo #311,
Office 740
Borough: Colonia Fracción del Cerro Gordo
Work/Fax: (477) 788-5674
Home: (477) 717-0685
Mobile: 044-477-147-0911
Nextel: 34656*6
Email: funrpp@prodigy.net.mx

IMMUNOLOGIST

Dr. Carlos Ramírez-Mateos
Internal Medicine, Hematology, Immunology
Address: Avenida Cerro Gordo #311,
Office 740
Borough: Colonia Fracción del Cerro Gordo
Work/Fax: (477) 788-5674
Home: (477) 717-0685
Mobile: 044-477-147-0911
Nextel: 34656*6
Email: funrpp@prodigy.net.mx

INTERNISTS

Dr. Carlos Harrison
Internal Medicine, Cardiology, Critical Care
Address: Avenida Cerro Gordo #311,
Office 910
Borough: Colonia Fracción del Cerro Gordo
Work/Fax: (477) 788-5691
Mobile: 044-477-638-5954
Pager: 01-800-500-1212, PIN #4776385954
Email: charrison@angelesleon.com

Dr. Carlos Ramírez-Mateos
Internal Medicine, Hematology, Immunology
Address: Avenida Cerro Gordo #311,
Office 740
Borough: Colonia Fracción del Cerro Gordo
Work/Fax: (477) 788-5674
Home: (477) 717-0685
Mobile: 044-477-147-0911
Nextel: 34656*6
Email: funrpp@prodigy.net.mx

NEONATOLOGISTS

Dr. David González-Flores
Pediatrics, Neonatology
Address: Avenida Cerro Gordo #311,
Office 120
Borough: Colonia Fracción del Cerro Gordo
Work/Fax: (477) 788-5612, 143-9291
Mobile: 044-477-724-9103
Nextel: 177563*2

Email: gfdavid02@yahoo.com.mx,
gfdavid@angelesleon.com

OBSTETRICIANS

Dr. Héctor López-Frisbie
Obstetrics & Gynecology
Address: Avenida Cerro Gordo #311,
Office 210
Borough: Colonia Fracción del Cerro Gordo
Work: (477) 788-5621, 788-5721
Home: (477) 781-1668
Mobile: 044-477-159-3333
Nextel: 177413*1
Email: drlopezfrisbie@gmail.com

Dra. Sara Gutiérrez
Obstetrics & Gynecology, Gynecologic
Urology
Address: Plaza de las Américas #115
Borough: Colonia Jardines del Moral
Work/Fax: (477) 714-2139, 779-0608
Pager: (477) 714-8022, PIN# 700496
Email: sgtct@hotmail.com

OPHTALMOLOGISTS

Dr. Luis A. Alanís
Ophthalmology, Corneal and Refractive
Surgery
Address: Avenida Cerro Gordo #311,
Office 510 (in Front of the Plaza Mayor)
Borough: Colonia Fracción del Cerro Gordo
Work: (477) 788-5633
Fax: (477) 788-5633, ext. 1
Toll Free: 01-800-836-2436
Email: luis-alanis@angelesleon.com

ORTHOPEDICS / TRAUMATOLOGY

Dr. Roberto Méndez
Orthopedics and Traumatology, sub-specialty in
Hip Surgery
Address: Avenida Hidalgo #327, 3rd floor,

Office 302
Work: (477) 716-9614
Home: (477) 717-1240
Pager: (477) 714-8022, PIN# 755236
Email:
dr.robertomendezfernandez@hotmail.com

PEDIATRICIANS

Dr. David González-Flores
Pediatrics, Neonatology
Address: Avenida Cerro Gordo #311,
Office 120
Borough: Colonia Fracción del Cerro Gordo
Work/Fax: (477) 788-5612, 143-9291
Mobile: 044-477-724-9103
Nextel: 177563*2
Email: gfdavid02@yahoo.com.mx,
gfdavid@angelesleon.com

SURGEONS

Dr. Ernesto Marín
General Surgery, Gastroenterology
Address: Avenida Cerro Gordo #311,
Office 610
Borough: Colonia Fracción del Cerro Gordo
Work: (477) 788-5661
Home: (477) 781-0669
Mobile: 044-477-729-1343
Email: emarin@angelesleon.com

HOSPITALS

Hospital Angeles – León
Address: Avenida Cerro Gordo, #311
(at the corner of Boulevard López Sanabria)
Borough: Colonia Fracción del Cerro Gordo
Notable Landmarks:
In front of the Plaza Mayor
Main Phone: (477) 788-5600, 788-5700
Fax Phone: (477) 788-5600, ext. 2001
Emergency Phone: (477) 788-5600, ext. 2105

Hospital Aranda de la Parra
Address: Calle Hidalgo #329

Borough: Centro Histórico
Notable Landmarks: near the Casa Municipal
Main Phone: (477) 719-7100
Fax Phone: (477) 716-4903
Emergency Phone #: (477) 719-7101
Administrative Contact: Víctor Mancilla
Office Phone #: (477) 719-7100, ext. 126
Fax Phone #: (477) 716-4903
Email: direccion@arandadelaparra.com

LORETO

Clínica del ISSTE
Calle Tamaral (no street number)
Colonia Centro
Loreto, Baja California Sur
Tel: (613) 135-0730 / 135-0345

Unidad de Medicina Familiar
Calle Pedro Ugarte entre Francisco Barnes (no street number)
Loreto B.C.S.
Tel: (613) 135-0730

MANZANILLO

AMBULANCES

Centro Médico Echauri
Dr. Edmundo Echauri Fletes
Blvd. Miguel De La Madrid Km 9.7
Col. Salahua, Manzanillo, Colima
Tel: (314) 334-0001 / 1666
Tel. & Fax: (314) 334-0444

Cruz Roja Mexicana
Avenida Parotas on the corner of Cedro
Fracc. Valle de las Garzas
Manzanillo, Colima

Tel: (314) 336-5770
Emergencies (dialling from Manzanillo only): 065
(only spanish spoken)

Médica Pacífico
Dr. Jorge Alvarado Pérez
Avenida Palma Real 10
Col. Salahua, Manzanillo, Colima
Tel: (314) 334-0385
Fax: (314) 334-1828
Cell: (314) 353-0110

GENERAL MEDICINE

Dr. Sergio Arranguré Lizarraga
Hotel Las Hadas
Colonia La Audiencia
Manzanillo, Colima
Tel.: (314) 331-0101
Cell: (314) 116-9100

Dr. Jorge Bernardino Alvarado
Av. Palma Real 10
Colonia Salahua
Manzanillo, Colima
Tel.: (314) 334-0385 / 333-3047
Cell: (314) 358-0100
E-mail: medicapacifico@hotmail.com

CARDIOLOGISTS

Dr. Martin Toscano Ramírez
Centro Médico Echauri
Boulevard Costero Miguel De La Madrid 1215
Colonia Salahua
Manzanillo, Colima
Tel.: (314) 334-1666 / 334-0444

DENTISTS

Dr. Jesús Ibarra Rojas
Dental Surgery
75 Av. Elias Zamora Verduzco 151 L-11
Valle de las Garzas
Manzanillo, Colima

Tel.: (314) 334-2565
E-mail: odent_manzanillo@yahoo.com.mx

Dr. Salvador Salcedo Solís
Emiliano Zapata 2
Crucero de Las Brisas
Manzanillo, Colima
Tel.: (314) 334-2599
E-mail: annapvl@hotmail.com

DIABETES

Dr. Ariel Gutiérrez-Aparicio
Internal Medicine, Diabetes
Address: Boulevard Miguel de la Madrid 1215
Work: (314) 334-0001, 334-0444, 334-2160
Mobile: 044-314-305-0190
Email: aga20@prodigy.net.com.mx

EAR, NOSE & THROAT

Dr. Daniel Macías Ramirez
Centro Médico Echauri
Boulevard Costero Miguel De La Madrid 1215
Colonia Salahua
Manzanillo, Colima
Tel.: (314) 334-1666 / 334-0444

GASTROENTEROLOGISTS

Dr. Julio César Martinez Salgado
Centro Médico Echauri
Boulevard Costero Miguel De La Madrid 1215
Colonia Salahua
Manzanillo, Colima
Tel.: (314) 334-1666 / 334-0444

GYNECOLOGISTS

Dra. Beatriz Aranzolo Tejeda
Centro Médico Echauri
Boulevard Costero Miguel De La Madrid 1215
Colonia Salahua
Manzanillo, Colima
Tel.: (314) 334-1666 / 334-0444

Dr. Luis Angel De La Torre
Centro Médico Echauri
Boulevard Costero Miguel De La Madrid 1215
Colonia Salahua
Manzanillo, Colima
Tel.: (314) 334-1666 / 334-0444

Dr. Carlos Hernández
Centro Médico Echauri
Boulevard Costero Miguel De La Madrid 1215
Colonia Salahua
Manzanillo, Colima
Tel.: (314) 334-1666 / 334-0444

Dr. César G. Ruíz-García
Obstetrics & Gynecology
Address: Boulevard Miguel de la Madrid 444
Work: (314) 336-4225, 336-7272, 336-7273
Home: (314) 335-0229
Mobile: 044-314-358-0364
Email: seaczar@prodigy.net.mx

INTERNISTS

Dra. Erika Echauri Marroquin
Centro Médico Echauri
Boulevard Costero Miguel De La Madrid 1215
Colonia Salahua
Manzanillo, Colima
Tel.: (314) 334-1666 / 334-0444
Cell: (314) 358-6969

Dr. Ariel Gutiérrez Aparicio
Centro Médico Echauri
Boulevard Costero Miguel De La Madrid 1215
Colonia Salahua
Manzanillo, Colima
Tel.: (314) 334-1666 / 334-0444 / 334-0001/
334-2160
Cell: (314) 305-0190
E-mail: aga20@prodigy.net.mx

Dr. René Pantoja
Centro Médico Echauri
Boulevard Costero Miguel De La Madrid 1215
Colonia Salahua
Manzanillo, Colima
Tel.: (314) 334-1666 / 334-0444

NEPHROLOGISTS

Dr. J. Jesús Venegas Ramirez
Centro Médico Echauri
Blvd Costero Miguel De La Madrid 1215
Colonia Salahua
Manzanillo, Colima
Tel.: (314) 334-1666 / 334-0444
E-mail: emodialisismanzanillo@hotmail.com

OBSTETRICIANS

Dr. César G. Ruíz-García
Obstetrics & Gynecology
Address: Boulevard Miguel de la Madrid 444
Work: (314) 336-4225, 336-7272, 336-7273
Home: (314) 335-0229
Mobile: 044-314-358-0364
Email: seaczar@prodigy.net.mx

ORTHOPEDISTS

Dr. Edmundo Echauri Fletes
Centro Médico Echauri
Boulevard Costero Miguel De La Madrid 1215
Colonia Salahua, Manzanillo, Colima
Tel.: (314) 334-1666 / 334-0444 / 334-2696
E-mail: edmundoef44@hotmail.com

Dr. Edmundo Echauri Marroquin
Centro Médico Echauri
Boulevard Costero Miguel De La Madrid 1215
Colonia Salahua, Manzanillo, Colima
Tel.: (314) 334-1666 / 334-0444 / 334-2696

PEDIATRICIANS

Dr. Raúl González Sánchez
Centro Médico Echauri
Boulevard Costero Miguel De La Madrid 1215
Colonia Salahua
Manzanillo, Colima
Tel.: (314) 334-1666 / 334-0444

Dr. Jaime Virgen Perez
Centro Médico Echauri

Boulevard Costero Miguel De La Madrid 1215
Colonia Salahua
Manzanillo, Colima
Tel.: (314) 334-1666 / 334-0444

PSYCHIATRIST

Dr. Javier Hernández
Unidad Psiquiátrica Hospital Manzanillo
Blvd Miguel De La Madrid 444
Fondeport
Manzanillo, Colima
Tel.: (314) 336-7272

UROLOGISTS

Dr. Julio Háctor Bedolla
Centro Médico Echauri
Boulevard Costero Miguel De La Madrid 1215
Colonia Salahua, Manzanillo, Colima
Tel: (314) 334-1666 / 334-0444 / 334-2500
E-mail: bedollajh@hotmail.com

HOSPITALS

Centro Médico Echauri (Private)
Boulevard Costero Miguel De La Madrid 1215
Colonia Salahua, Manzanillo, Colima
Tel.: (314) 334-1666 / 334-0444
Fax: (314) 332-0761
E-mail: cmechauri@gmail.com

Centro Médico Quirúrgico Echauri
Address: Boulevard Miguel de la Madrid 1215
Borough: Colonia Salagua
Notable Landmarks: Near Manzanillo Bay, Comercial Mexicana, in front of the VW agency
Main Phone #: (314) 334-0444, 334-1666
Fax Phone #: (314) 334-0444, ext. 102
Emergency Phone #: (314) 334-0444, ext. 122

Hospital Civil Manzanillo (Public)
Avenida Elias Zamora Verduzco 1500
Colonia Arboledas, Manzanillo, Colima
Tel.: (314) 332-0029

Hospital General de Manzanillo (Public)
Calle Hospital (no street number)
Manzanillo, Colima
Tel.: (314) 332-1903

Hospital Manzanillo
Blvd. Miguel de la Madrid 444
Tel. (314) 336-7272 & (314) 336-7273
Manzanillo, Colima

Hospital Médica Pacífico (Private)
Avenida Palma Real 10
Colonia Salahua
Manzanillo, Colima
Tel.: (314) 333-3047 / 334-0385
Enail: dralvarado@medicapacifico.com

MATAMOROS

DENTISTS

Dr. Ceferino Aldrete Torres,
Ave. Alvaro Obregón #34, Colonia Jardín
Entre Claveles y Segunda.
H. Matamoros, Tamaulipas
Office hours: 9 am to 1 pm & 3 pm to 7 pm
Tel & Fax: (868) 813 43 60
Universidad Autónoma de Nuevo León
Thirty-five years of experience.

Dr. Ricardo Diaz Garza Jr.,
Specializing in: Orthodontics
Margaritas # 20
entre Colegio Militar y Claveles,
Colonia Jardín, H. Matamoros, Tamaulipas
Office hours: 8:30am to 1pm & 2pm to 7pm
Monday–Friday, 7:30am to 2:30pm Saturdays
Tel: (868) 813 13 01
Fax: (868) 813 07 61
E-mail: ricdiazg@aol.com
Universidad Autónoma de Nuevo León
and the Charles H. Tweed Institute in
Tucson, Arizona.

Twenty-nine years of experience.
Member of the American
Association of Orthodontists.

Dr. Rubén Alberto Martínez Córdova,
Specializing in: Endodontics
Alhelies # 46, Colonia Jardín
H. Matamoros, Tamaulipas
Office hours: 9 am to 6 pm Monday–Friday
and 9 am to 2 pm Saturdays
Tel & Fax: (868) 812 14 64
Cell: (956) 793 66 59
E-mail: alhelies46@yahoo.com
Universidad Autónoma de Nuevo León
Eighteen years of experience.

EAR, NOSE & THROAT

Dr. Gregorio Francisco Hernández Beltran,
Specializing in: Otorhinolaryngology
Calle Amapolas entre 1 y 2 #16,
Colonia Jardín
Office hours: 9 am to 2 pm & 4 pm to 8 pm
Tel: (868) 816 22 60
Fax: (868) 816 22 61
E-mail: pacootorrino@yahoo.com
Universidad Autónoma de Tamaulipas y
Centro Médico del Noreste Monterrey, N.L.
Twenty-six years of experience.

Dr. Ignacio Mendoza Hernández,
Specializing in: Otorhinolaryngology,
allergies, ear, nose and throat.
Calle Bustamante entre 4a y 5a, No. 405 Zona
Centro
Office hours: 9 am to 1 pm & 4 pm to 7 pm
Monday–Friday, 9 am to 1 pm Saturdays
Tel & Fax: (868) 811-0010
E-mail: imendoza56@yahoo.com.mx
Universidad Autónoma de Tamaulipas,
Clinic "Trabajo de la Seguridad Social" in
Madrid, Spain, and Resource Fellowship
Otoneurology "Ear International" in Los
Angeles, CA.
Twenty three years of experience.

GASTROENTEROLOGISTS

Dr. Carlos Jaime Aguirre Martínez,
Specializing in: Gastroenterology, General Surgery (surgical oncology) and Laparoscopy
Calle Sexta entre Rayón y Victoria # 72,
Zona Centro
Office hours: 11 am to 2 pm & 6 pm to 9 pm, 11 am to 2 pm Saturdays
Tel & Fax: (868) 816 71 81
E-mail: caja58@prodigy.net.mx
Universidad Autónoma de Tamaulipas,
Universidad Nacional Autónoma de
México, Centro Médico Nacional Siglo XXI.
Twenty years of experience. 4

Dr. José Benjamín Pérez Alonso,
Specializing in: Gastroenterology and
General Surgery
Calle Primera entre Ocampo y Mina # 213,
Zona Centro
Office hours: 9 am to 2 pm & 4 pm to 8 pm
Tel: (868) 8 13 22 70
E-mail: bepa50@yahoo.com
Universidad Nacional Autónoma de México and
Secretaria de Salubridad y Asistencia
Thirty-four years of experience.

Dr. Hugo Torres Díaz,
Specializing in: Gastroenterology and
General Surgery
Calle González Entre 1 y 2 #134,
Zona Centro
Office hours: 10 am to 6 pm
Tel: (868) 813 43 94
Fax: (868) 813 15 15
E-mail: htorrespuma@hotmail.com
Universidad Nacional Autónoma de México and
Centro Médico Nacional del Instituto Mexicano del Seguro Social, Mexico, DF.
Thirty-eighteen years of experience.

GENERAL SURGEONS

Dr. José Eugenio Najera Lozano,
Specializing in: General Surgery and
Gastroenterology

Victoria entre 5a y 6a #502 Esquina,
Zona Centro
Office hours: 11 am to 1 pm & 4 pm to 7 pm
Monday–Friday, 9 am to 1 pm Saturday
Tel: (868) 8 16 10 94 and 813 94 15
Fax: (868) 8 16 49 98
E-mail: eugenionajeralozano@hotmail.com
Universidad Autónoma de Tamaulipas,
Universidad de Monterrey
Twenty four years of experience.

Dr. Cuauhtémoc Ramírez Cadena,
Specializing in: General Surgery and
Phlebology
Calle Sexta entre Mina y Ocampo #205,
Zona Centro
Office hours: 10 am to 2 pm & 5 pm to 8 pm
Monday–Friday
Tel: (868) 8 16 52 32
Fax: (868) 8 16 55 88
E-mail: cuauhtemoc57@hotmail.com

GYNECOLOGISTS / OBSTETRICIAN

Dr. Jesús Martínez Castañeda,
Specializing in: Gynecology & Obstetrics, Laparoscopy and Fertility Specialist
Prolongación Francisco Villa y Luis Pasteur (no street number), Colonia Doctores
Office hours: 9 am to 1 pm & 4 pm to 8 pm
Monday–Friday, 9 am to 2 pm Saturdays
Tel: (868) 810 7373
Fax: (868) 812 5345
Email: drmartinezcj@hotmail.com
Universidad Autónoma de Tamaulipas and
Instituto de Ciencias en Reproducción
Humana de Guadalajara.
Five years of experience.

Dr. Gabriel Martínez Del Bosque,
Specializing in: Gynecology & Obstetrics Calle Sexta Rayón y Victoria # 72,
Zona Centro
Office hours: 4 pm to 8 pm Monday–Friday, 10 am to 1 pm Saturdays

Tel & Fax: (868) 813 94 15
Email: gobidels08@live.com.mx
Universidad Autónoma de Tamaulipas
Twelve years of experience.

INTERNISTS

Dr. René Cuellar Garza,
Specializing in: Family Medicine
Luis Pasteur on the corner of (no street number), Colonia Doctores
Office hours: 9 am to 1:30 pm & 5 pm to 8 pm
Monday–Friday, 9 am to 2 pm Saturdays
Tel & Fax: (868) 810 73 73
Universidad de Monterrey y Universidad Nacional Autónoma de México
Thirty years of experience.

Dr. Horacio Ramírez Oropeza,
Calle González 1 y 2 #134, Zona Centro
Office hours: 11 am to 2 pm & 5 pm to 8 pm
Monday–Friday
Tel: (868) 812 31 29
Fax: (868) 813 15 15
E-mail: hramirezo@hotmail.com
Specializing in: Internal Medicine
Universidad Nacional Autónoma de México
& I.M.S.S.
Forty years of experience.

Dr. Gerardo Rosario Zúñiga Quintanilla,
Calle Victoria 5a y 6a #502, Zona Centro
Office hours: 3 pm to 10 pm
Tel: (868) 813 55 71
Fax: (868) 816 10 82
E-mail: gerry_2_2@hotmail.com
Specializing in: General Medicine
Universidad Autónoma de Tamaulipas
Twenty-one years of experience.

ORTHOPEDICS / TRAUMATOLOGISTS

Dr. José Lara Esquivel,
Orthopedist and Traumatologist
Calle Sexta # 72, Entre Rayón y Victoria

Office hours: 5 pm to 8 pm Monday–Friday
Tel & Fax: (868) 8 16 10 82
Universidad Autónoma de Nuevo León, I.M.S.S.
Eighteen years of experience.

Dr. Alfonso Hector Leal Ammler,
Specializing in: Orthopedics and
Traumatologist
Calle Amapolas # 5, Col. Jardín
Office hours: 10 am to 1 pm & 5 pm to 7 pm
Monday–Friday, 10 am to 1 pm Saturdays
Tel : (868) 8 12 22 26
Fax: (868) 8 12 22 09
E-mail: lealammler@hotmail.com
Universidad Autónoma de Nuevo León
and Centro Médico Del Noreste I.M.S.S.
Twenty three years of experience. 7

PEDIATRICIANS

Solis Fernandez, Juventino
Calle Sexta # 72 Norte, Entre Rayón y
Victoria, Zona Centro
Office hours: 10 am to 2 pm & 5 pm to 9 pm
Monday–Friday
Tel: (868) 8 13 95 17
Fax: (868) 8 16 10 82
E-mail: drjuvesolis@hotmail.com
Specializing in: Pediatrician
Univerisidad Autónoma de Nuevo León
and Hospital Universitario "Dr. José E.
González" UANL
Twenty-five years of experience.

RADIOLOGISTS

Dr. Sergio Antonio Novelo Tello,
Calle General González No. 18
entre 1 y 2, Zona Centro
Office hours: 9 am to 3 pm Monday–Friday
Tel: (868) 8 16 23 62
Fax: (868) 8 12 08 81
Email: arsaar@hotmail.com
Specializing in: Radiology and Ultrasound
Universidad Nacional Autónoma de México and
Hospital "20 de Noviembre", México City.
Thirty-eight years of experience.

HOSPITALS

Centro de Especialidades Medico Quirurgicas
Calle 1a y Gonzalez Esquina,
Zona Centro
Tel: (868) 813 43 03

Clinica de Leon y Garza
Amapolas #5 entre 1a y 2a,
Colonia Jardín
Tel: (868) 8 12 15 20, 8 12 15 21,
8 12 15 22 & 8 12 15 23
Fax: (868) 8 12 60 10
E-mail: clinicaleonygarza@hotmail.com

Centro de Salud
Sexta y Queretaro (no street number),
Col/ Euzcadi
Tel: (868) 819-16 20

Clinica Hospital AmE.
Ave. Lauro Villar No. 102, Colonia Modelo
Tel: (868) 8 16 39 27, 8 16 38 74 &
8 13 69 89
Fax: ext. 122

Clinica Hospital Guadalupe
Calle 6a #72 entre Rayon y Victoria
Tel: (868) 8 13 94 15, 8 13 95 17,
8 13 96 76 & 8 12 16 55
Fax: (868) 8 16 10 82

Clinica Hospital San Francisco
14th y Paseo de la Reforma,
(on the corner of)
Colonia San Francisco
Tel: (868) 8 16 61 10 & 8 16 61 11

Centro Medico Internacional
Av. Longoria #9,
Fraccionamiento Victoria, Sección Fiesta
Tel: (868) 811 00 50
www.cmi-matamoros.com

Laboratorios "Uni-Lab"
Calle No. 614, 7 entre Rayón y Zaragoza
Office Hours: 7 am to 8 pm & 7 am to 1 pm
Monday–Friday
Tel: (868) 8 16 59 99

MATEHUALA

HOSPITALS

Hospital General de Matehuala
Ave. Miguel Hidalgo Norte # 200,
Col. Centro
Matehuala, San Luis Potosí,
Tel (488) 882-0445
Fax (488) 882-4488

Hospital Rural No 14 de Oportunidades IMSS
Carretera Central Km. 617
(Frente al Hotel Las Palmas)
Matehuala, San Luis Potosí
Teléfono (488) 882-0152

MAZATLAN

GENERAL PHYSICIANS

Dra. Adriana Montes
Mariano Ramos 127, El Toreo
Mazatlán, Sinaloa
Tel: (669) 986-7357
E-mail: dradmon@hotmail.com

Dr. Miguel Angel Guzman
Guillermo Nelson 1808
Col. Centro
Mazatlán, Sinaloa
Tel/Fax: (669) 981-2587
E-mail: ma_g_elizondomd@hotmail.com

CARDIOLOGISTS

Dr. Miguel Ángel Morales Barraza
Polimédica Sharp Hospital
Ave. Rafael Buelna 198, 3rd floor, Office 319

Fracc. Hacienda Las Cruces
Mazatlán, Sinaloa
Tel: (669) 984-6604 / 984-2999
E-mail: mmorales@hotmail.com

Dr. Jorge M. Valdés
Internal Medicine, Cardiology
Address: Avenida Revolución #5
Borough: Colonia López Mateos
Work: (669) 986-7618
Home: (669) 913-2251
Mobile: 044-669-918-2782

DENTISTS

Dra. Paty Ascencio D.D.S.
Alameda Shopping Center
Ave. Camaron Sabalo 1502-8
Sabalo Country
Mazatlán, Sinaloa
Tel: (669) 668-0548
E-mail: patydds@yahoo.com.mx

Dr. Arturo Humberto Barros de Cima
Rio San Lorenzo 220-D
Colonia Palos Prietos
Mazatlán, Sinaloa
Tel: (669) 982-0215
E-mail: arturobarros@hotmail.com

Dr. Juan Jaime Diaz Rivas
Universidad Autónoma de Guadalajara
Ave. Rafael Buelna 202 local 10
Plaza Las Conchas (frente a Hospital Sharp)
Hacienda las Cruces
Mazatlán, Sinaloa
Tel: (669) 983-3300
Cell: (669) 918-2442
E-mail: jjaimedr63@hotmail.com /
jjaimedr63@yahoo.com.mx
Website: www.drjaimediaz.com

Dr. César Gavito
Av. Camarón Sábalo 51, Office 8
Zona Dorada
Mazatlán, Sinaloa
Tel: (669) 984-1850
E-mail: cesargavito@prodigy.net.mx

Dr. Jorge Morelos Chong
Centro Comercial Las Lomas
Av. Camarón Sábalo 204, 2nd floor,
Office 30, Zona Dorada
Mazatlán, Sinaloa
Tel: (669) 913-6068
E-mail: morelos@mzt.megared.net.mx

DENTISTS

Dra. Claudia Peniche
Specialty: Pediatric Dentistry
Calle 5 de Mayo 1725, 2nd floor,
Office 4
Col. Centro
Mazatlán, Sinaloa
Tel: (669) 981-5775 / 981-5022
E-mail: draclaudiapeniche@yahoo.com

EAR, NOSE & THROAT

Dr. René Contreras
Polimédica Sharp Hospital
Av. Rafael Buelna 198, 6th floor,
Office 605
Fracc. Hacienda Las Cruces
Mazatlán, Sinaloa
Tel: (669) 990-2857
Cell: (669) 901-3538
E-mail: contrerasvrene@hotmail.com

Dr. Israel Lizárraga Padilla
Polimédica Sharp Hospital
Av. Rafael Buelna 198,
Office 501
Fracc. Hacienda Las Cruces
Mazatlán, Sinaloa
Tel: (669) 112-0588 / 984-2923
Cell: (669) 132-1522
E-mail: israelpuntodoc@hotmail.com

ENDOCRINOLOGISTS

Dr. Rodolfo Rosas
Internal Medicine, Endocrinology
Address: Avenida Revolución #5

(corner of Insurgentes)
Borough: Colonia López Mateos
Work/Fax: (669) 983-8888
Home: (669) 913-4545
Mobile: 044-669-933-5687

ENDOSCOPIST

Dr. Elías A. Javer
Gastroenterology, Endoscopy
Address: Corner of Avenida Rafael Buelna and
Dr. Jesús Kumate, Office #308
Borough: Fraccionamiento Las Cruces
Work/Fax: (669) 984-2484
Mobile: 044-669-918-0460
Email: eliasjaver@hotmail.com

GASTROENTEROLOGISTS

Dr. Elías A. Javer
Gastroenterology, Endoscopy
Address: Corner of Avenida Rafael Buelna and
Dr. Jesús Kumate,
Office #308
Borough: Fraccionamiento Las Cruces
Work/Fax: (669) 984-2484
Mobile: 044-669-918-0460
Email: eliasjaver@hotmail.com

GYNECOLOGISTS

Dr. Alberto E. Donnadieu
Obstetrics & Gynecology
Address: Avenida Carnaval #1611,
Office 3
Work: (669) 982-0186
Fax: (669) 982-2597
Home: (669) 916-0991
Mobile: 044-669-918-0954
Email: aedonnadieu@hotmail.com

Dr. Jorge E. Montoya
Obstetrics & Gynecology
Address: Avenida Rafael Buelna #198,
Office 306, Polimédica building
Work: (669) 990-1904, 990-1919

Fax: (669) 990-1920
Home: (669) 914-4141
Mobile: 044-669-918-1737
Email: drjmontoya@hotmail.com

HEMATOLOGISTS

Dr. José de Jesús Ibarra
Internal Medicine, Hematology
Address: Avenida Ejército Mexicano #204-2
Borough: Colonia Palos Prietos
Work/Fax: (669) 985-1221
Home: (669) 914-0417
Mobile: 044-669-115-5079,
044-669-942-8257
Email: dr_jibarra@hotmail.com

INTERNISTS

Dr. José de Jesús Ibarra
Internal Medicine, Hematology
Address: Avenida Ejército Mexicano #204-2
Borough: Colonia Palos Prietos
Work/Fax: (669) 985-1221
Home: (669) 914-0417
Mobile: 044-669-115-5079,
044-669-942-8257
Email: dr_jibarra@hotmail.com

Dr. Rodolfo Rosas
Internal Medicine, Endocrinology
Address: Avenida Revolución #5
(corner of Insurgentes)
Borough: Colonia López Mateos
Work/Fax: (669) 983-8888
Home: (669) 913-4545
Mobile: 044-669-933-5687

Dr. Jorge M. Valdés
Internal Medicine, Cardiology
Address: Avenida Revolución #5
Borough: Colonia López Mateos
Work: (669) 986-7618
Home: (669) 913-2251
Mobile: 044-669-918-2782

NEUROLOGISTS

Dr. Alfredo Román Messina
Clínica del Mar
Ave. Revolución 5
Col. López Mateos
Mazatlán, Sinaloa
Tel: (669) 983-1524
Fax: (669) 983-1777
E-mail: arome@clinicadelmar.com.mx

OBSTETRICIAN

Dr. Alberto E. Donnadieu
Obstetrics & Gynecology
Address: Avenida Carnaval #1611,
Office 3
Work: (669) 982-0186
Fax: (669) 982-2597
Home: (669) 916-0991
Mobile: 044-669-918-0954
Email: aedonnadieu@hotmail.com

Dr. Jorge E. Montoya
Obstetrics & Gynecology
Address: Avenida Rafael Buelna #198,
Office 306, Polimédica building
Work: (669) 990-1904, 990-1919
Fax: (669) 990-1920
Home: (669) 914-4141
Mobile: 044-669-918-1737
Email: drjmontoya@hotmail.com

OPHTHALMOLOGISTS

Dr. Víctor Sánchez Malof
Clínica Del Mar
Ave. Revolución 5
Col. López Mateos
Mazatlán, Sinaloa
Tel/Fax: (669) 986-6401 / 983-3112
E-mail: vsanchezmalof@yahoo.com

ORTHOPEDISTS / TRAUMATOLOGISTS

Dr. José Luis Olmeda
Orthopedics/Traumatology
Address: Avenida Rafael Buelna #202,
Offices 11 & 12, Plaza Las Conchas
Work/Fax: (669) 983-0304
Mobile: 044-669-994-7621
Email: olmedamd@hotmail.com

Dr. Dagoberto Ramírez Gutiérrez
Clínica del Mar
Ave. Revolución 5
Col. López Mateos
Mazatlán, Sinaloa
Tel: (669) 990-1060
Fax: (669) 983-1777
E-mail: dagobertoramirezg@hotmail.com

PEDIATRICIANS

Dra. Claudia Vega
Ave. Lola Beltrán 211-D
Palos Prietos
Mazatlán, Sinaloa
Tel: (669) 985-2424
E-mail: claudia.vega@mamapediatra.com

SURGEON

Dr. Miguel A. Guzmán
General Surgery
Address: Calle Guillermo Nelson #1808
Borough: Colonia Centro (near the cathedral)
Work: (669) 981-2587
Fax: (669) 981-2164
Home: (669) 981-5117
Mobile: 044-669-918-1070
Email: miguel@mzt.megared.net.mx

HOSPITALS

Central Médica Quirúrgica
Ave. Ejército Mexicano 2207
Palos Prieto

Mazatlán, Sinaloa
Tel: (669) 985-0730 / 0997
E-mail: cemeq.admon@hotmail.com

Clínica del Mar
Address: Corner of Avenida Revolución
and Calle General Cabanillas
Borough: Colonia López Mateos
Main Phone: (669) 983-1777, 983-4238,
983-1524, 983-1958
Fax Phone: (669) 986-7254
E-mail: clidemar@prodigy.net.mx

Clínica San José
Alejandro Quijano 1403
Col. Centro
Mazatlán, Sinaloa
Tel: (669) 981-5008, 985-3670
Fax: (669) 981-5008
E-mail: pepehuizar@msn.com

Clínica Siglo XXI
Belisario Domínguez 2303
Col. Centro
Mazatlán, Sinaloa
Tel: (669) 985-5418 / 982-8310
Fax: (669) 985-2788
E-mail: sigloxx1@red2000.com.mx

Cruz Roja
Ave. Ignacio Zaragoza 1801
Col. Centro
Mazatlán, Sinaloa
Tel: (669) 985-1451
Emergencies: (669) 981-3690
Fax: (669) 985-2445
E-mail: cruzroja@red2000.com.mx

Hospital General
Ave. Americas and Ferrocarril
(no street number)
Col. Sta. Elena, Mazatlán, Sinaloa
Tel: (669) 984-0246
Fax: (669) 984-0233
E-mail: hg_mazatlan@hotmail.com

Hospital Militar Regional
Venus 1
Col. Centro,Mazatlán, Sinaloa,
Tel: (669) 981-2079 / 6033
Fax: (669) 981-2079

Hospital Sharp Mazatlán
Address: On Avenida Rafael Buelna
(corner of Avenida Dr. Jesús Kumate,
no street number)
Borough: Fraccionamiento Las Cruces
Notable Landmarks:
Visible from Avenida del Mar
Main Phone: (669) 986-5678, 986-5679,
986-5680/81/82/83/84
Fax Phone: (669) 986-5678, ext.108
Emergency Phone: (669) 986-7911
E-mail: info@hospitalsharp.com.mx

Sanatorio Divina Providencia
Galeana 619
Col. Centro, Mazatlán, Sinaloa
Tel: (669) 982-4011
Fax: (669) 982-3836
E-mail: terras06@hotmail.com

Sanatorio Mazatlán
Héctor González Guevara 1
Col. Centro, Mazatlán, Sinaloa
Tel: (669) 981-2508, 985-1097
Fax: (669) 985-2908
E-mail: mcp_41@hotmail.com

OXYGEN PROVIDERS

Oxigeno Medicinal
Puerto de Ensenada Lote 3 Mza. 5
Parque Industrial Bonfil
Mazatlán Sinaloa
Tel: (669) 981-3294 / 3429
E-mail: mazatlan@infra.com.mx
Website: www.inframedica.com

Praxair
Puerto de Veracruz 1
Parque Industrial Bonfil
Mazatlán Sinaloa
Tel: (669) 118-0823 to 25
E-mail: lino.gonzalez@praxair.com

MERIDA

ALLERGISTS

Dr. Jorge Carlos Bolaños Ancona,
Clinica de Merida, Av. Itzaes No. 242.
Col. Garcia Gineres, Merida, Yuc.
Tel: 925-8385

CARDIOLOGISTS

Dr. David Arjona Canto,
Clinica de Merida, Av. Itzaes No. 242.
Col. Garcia Gineres, Merida, Yuc.
Tel: 925-4487

Dr. Julio I. Farjat
Internal Medicine, Cardiology
Address: Calle 54 #365, Office 109
Borough: Colonia Centro
Work/Fax: (999) 926-9965
Home: (999) 944-2760
Mobile: 044-999-949-1111
Email: juliofarjat@prodigy.net.mx

Dr. Joaquin Jimenez Noh,
Clinica de Merida, Av. Itzaes No. 242.
Col. Garcia Gineres, Merida, Yuc.
Tel: 925-4976

Dr. Salvador Padilla
Internal Medicine, Cardiology
Address: Calle 54, #365
(corner of Avenida Pérez Ponce)
Col. Centro, Merida,
Work: (999) 926-2367
Fax: (999) 981-0461, 926-4710
Mobile: 044-999-910-9729
Email: spadillam@prodigy.net.mx

Dr. Sergio A. Villareal Umana,
Edificio Anexo (Centro Medico las Americas)
Calle 54 No. 365, Por Av. Perez Ponce,

First Floor C Room 9
Col. Centro, Merida, Yuc.
Tel: 926-6348

Dr. Carlos Wabi Dogre,
Clinica de Merida, Av. Itzaes No. 242.
Col. Garcia Gineres, Merida, Yuc.
Tel: 925-6255

DENTISTS

Dr. Carlos Alayola Montañez
Orthodontics Specialist,
Calle 60 No. 387-B Por 43,
Col. Centro. Merida, Yuc.
Tel: 923-5380, 928-5939

Dr. Javier Cámara Patrón,
Calle 17 No. 170 Por 8 y 10.
Col. Garcia Gineres Merida, Yuc.
Tel: 925-3399

Dr. Rafael Alonso Dominguez,
Centro Estetico Odontologico Av.
Cupules No. 74. Por 6 Y 8
Col. Garcia Gineres, Merida
Tel: 920-2461

Dra. Ana Leticia Morales Vera,
Calle 6 No. 489 Por 17 Y 19.
Col. Garcia Gineres, Merida, Yuc..
Tel: 928-6810

Dr. Rolando Peniche Marcín,
Centro Medico las Americas.
Calle 54 No. 365,
Por Av. Perez Ponce,
Col. Centro, Merida, Yuc.
Tel: 926-4434

DERMATOLOGISTS

Dr. Roger Enrique Perez Perez,
Clinica de Merida,
Av. Itzaes No. 242.
Col. Garcia Gineres, Merida, Yuc.
Tel: 925-9976

Dr. María Rosa Rivero Vallado,
Clinica de Merida,
Av. Itzaes No. 242.
Col. Garcia Gineres, Merida, Yuc.
Tel: 925-8406

EAR, NOSE & THROAT

Dr. Miguel Baquedano Sauri,
Centro Especialidades Medicas,
Calle 60 No. 329-B Por 35 Y Av.
Colon, Merida, Yuc.
Tel: 925-5034

Dr. Juan José Castellanos Dorbecker,
Star Medica,
Calle 26 No. 199 x 15 x 7,
Fracc. Altabrisa. 728
Tel: 943-2991

Dr. Sergio Ivan Díaz Esquivel,
Centro Medico las Americas.
Calle 54 No. 365,
Por Av. Perez Ponce,
Col. Centro, Merida, Yuc.
Tel: 926-4278

EMERGENCIES

Dr. Juan José Falcón Arias,
Centro Especialidades Medicas,
Calle E 60 No. 329-B Por 3
Tel: 920-4040 ext 116
5 y Av. Colon, Merida, Yuc.

ENDOCRINOLOGISTS

Dr. Mario Barrero Estrada,
Centro Medico Pensiones,
Ave. Barrera Vazquez No. 215-A.
Col. Pensiones, Merida, Yuc.
Tel: 920-1037

Dr. Hugo Laviada Molina,
Clinica de Merida,
Av. Itzaes No. 242.

Col. Garcia Gineres, Merida, Yuc.
Tel: 925-8233

GASTROENTEROLOGISTS

Dr. Francisco Rivero Maldonado,
Clinica de Merida, Av.
Itzaes No. 242.
Col. Garcia Gineres, Merida, Yuc.
Tel: 925-4776
(Spanish only)

Dr. Tonatiuh Moreno Terrazas,
Specialist in Gastroenterology and
Laparoscopic Surgery
Sacbe Clinic,
Phone: 803-0055

GENERAL PRACTITIONERS

Dr. Humberto Angulo Cortes
Centro Medico las Americas.
Calle 54 No. 365,
Por Av. Perez Ponce,
Tel: 926-3078
Col. Centro, Merida, Yuc.

Dr. Eduardo Mena Arana,
Clinica de Merida, Av. Itzaes No. 242.
Col. Garcia Gineres, Merida, Yuc.
Tel: 925 8233
(Spanish only)

GENERAL SURGERY

Dr. Miguel Fernandez Martinez,
Star Medica,
Calle 26 No. 199 x 15 x 7,
Fracc. Altabrisa. 404
Tel: 943-7070

Dr. Luis Alberto Navarrete Jaimes,
Clinica de Merida,
Av. Itzaes No. 242.
Col. Garcia Gineres, Merida, Yuc.
Tel: 920-0949

GYNECOLOGISTS

Dr. Catalina Aldana de Mendez,
Star Medica,
Calle 26 No. 199 x 15 x 7,
Fracc. Altabrisa. 920
Tel: 943-2694

Dr. Manuel Mendez Arceo,
Star Medica,
Calle 26 No. 199 x 15 x 7,
Fracc. Altabrisa. 921
Tel: 943-1344

Dr. José A. Pereira Carcano
Obstetrics & Gynecology
Address: Avenida Itzaes, #242,
Office 315
Col. Garcia Gineres, Merida,
Work/Fax: (999) 925-8686, 925-6819

Dr. Luis Jesus Rodriguez Bolio,
Clinica de Merida,
Av. Itzaes No. 242.
Col. Garcia Gineres, Merida, Yuc.
Tel: 925-3998

INTERNISTS

Dr. Otto Bauerle
Internal Medicine, Respirology
Address: Calle 54 #365, Office 211
(at the corner of Avenida Pérez Ponce)
Work: (999) 926-9805
Mobile: 044-999-970-0552
Email: obauerle@yahoo.com

Dr. Antonio A. Briceño
Internal Medicine, Osteoporosis
Address: Avenida Itzaes, #242, Office #113
Col. Garcia Gineres, Merida,
Work: (999) 925-0868
Mobile: 044-999-947-7856
Email: drtony@sureste.com

Dr. Julio I. Farjat
Internal Medicine, Cardiology
Address: Calle 54 #365, Office 109
Borough: Colonia Centro
Work/Fax: (999) 926-9965
Home: (999) 944-2760
Mobile: 044-999-949-1111
Email: juliofarjat@prodigy.net.mx

Dr. Salvador Padilla
Internal Medicine, Cardiology
Address: Calle 54, #365
(corner of Avenida Pérez Ponce)
Col. Centro, Merida,
Work: (999) 926-2367
Fax: (999) 981-0461, 926-4710
Mobile: 044-999-910-9729
Email: spadillam@prodigy.net.mx

Dr. Sergio A. Villareal Umana,
Edificio Anexo (Centro Medico las Americas).
Calle 54 No. 365, Por Av. Perez Ponce,
First Floor C Room 9
Col. Centro, Merida,
Tel: 926-6348

NEUROLOGISTS

Dr. Ruben Dario Vargas García,
Clinica de Merida, Av. Itzaes No. 242.
Col. Garcia Gineres, Merida, Yuc.
Tel: 925-7508

OBSTETRICIANS

Dr. José A. Pereira Carcano
Obstetrics & Gynecology
Address: Avenida Itzaes, #242, Office 315
Col. Garcia Gineres, Merida, Yuc.
Work/Fax: (999) 925-8686, 925-6819

ONCOLOGISTS

Dr. Delio Ceballos Bojorquez,
Clinica de Merida,
Av. Itzaes No. 242.
Col. Garcia Gineres, Merida, Yuc.
Tel: 925-5499, 925-8333

OPHTHALMOLOGISTS

Dr. Adolfo Baqueiro Díaz,
Clinica de Merida,
Av. Itzaes No. 242.
Col. Garcia Gineres, Merida, Yuc.
Tel: 925-3253

Dr. Alberto Caceres Peniche,
Clinica de Merida,
Av. Itzaes No. 242.
Col. Garcia Gineres, Merida, Yuc.
Tel: 925-4152

Dr. Alejandro Millet Molina,
Clinica de Merida,
Av. Itzaes No. 242.
Col. Garcia Gineres, Merida, Yuc.
Tel: 925-6944

ORTHOPEDISTS

Dr. Luis Mario Baeza Mezquita,
Centro Medico las Americas.
Calle 54 No. 365,
Por Av. Perez Ponce,
Col. Centro, Merida, Yuc..
Tel: 926-2154

Dr. Felipe Eduardo Camara Arrigunaga,
Star Medica,
Calle 26 No. 199 x 15 x 7,
Fracc. Altabrisa. 928
Tel: 943-6202, 943-7202

Dr. Eduardo Muñoz Menendez,
Clinica de Merida,
Av. Itzaes No. 242.
Col. Garcia Gineres, Merida, Yuc.
Tel: 925-4865

Dr. Javier Pasos Novelo,
Centro Medico las Americas.
Calle 54 No. 365,
Por Av. Perez Ponce,
Col. Centro, Merida, Yuc..
Tel: 926-2009

Dr. Herbe Rivero Maldonado,
Clinica de Merida,
Av. Itzaes No. 242.
Col. Garcia Gineres,
Merida, Yuc.
Tel: 920-1658

PEDIATRICIANS

Dr. Gregorio Cetina Sauri,
Medica Itzaes Especialidades
Av. Itzaes No. 252 x 29,
Merida, Yuc.
Tel: 925-7056

Dr. Carlos Lara Navarrete,
Centro Medico las Americas.
Calle 54 No. 365,
Por Av. Perez Ponce,
Col. Centro, Merida, Yuc.
Tel: 926-2920

Dr. J. Enrique Ortegón Ruiz
Address: Avenida Itzaes, #242,
Office #2
Co. Garcia Gineres, Merida, Yuc.
Work: (999) 925-9944
Fax: (999) 925-9944
Home: (999) 925-1593
Mobile: 044-999-947-3032
Email: eortegon@prodigy.net.mx

PNEUMOLOGISTS

Dr. Nicolas Hernandez Flores,
Clinica de Merida,
Av. Itzaes No. 242.
Col. Garcia Gineres, Merida, Yuc.
Tel: 925-8218

Dr. Javier Torre Bolio,
Centro Medico las Americas.
Calle 54 No. 365,
Por Av. Perez Ponce,
Col. Centro, Merida, Yuc.
Tel: 926-8589

PSYCHIATRISTS

Dr. Roberto Carrillo Ruiz,
Calle 15 No. 251-1 x 36 x 38,
Fracc. Campestre, Merida, Yuc.
Tel: 944-7347

Dr. Arsenio Rosado Franco,
Av. Colon No. 199A x 24,
Col. Garcia Gineres, Merida, Yuc.
Tel: 920-1644

RESPIROLOGISTS

Dr. Otto Bauerle
Internal Medicine, Respirology
Address: Calle 54 #365, Office 211
(at the corner of Avenida Pérez Ponce)
Work: (999) 926-9805
Mobile: 044-999-970-0552
Email: obauerle@yahoo.com

SURGEONS

Dr. Martin Hernandez Lopez,
Medica del Carmen,
Phone: 873-0885

Dr. Salvador Martin Mandujano,
Costamed,
Phone: 807-7777

Dr. Fernando Moreno Polo,
Hospiten,
Phone: 803-1002

Dr. Tonatiuh Moreno Terrazas,
Specialist in Gastroenterology and
Laparoscopic Surgery
Sacbe Clinic,
Phone: 803-0055

Dr. Hector J. Perez Corzo,
Specializes in Gastric Bypass
Phone: 120-4400, 241-0980

Dr. Miguel Angel Rico Hinojosa,
Hospiten,

Phone: 803-1002

Dr. Ricardo Segovia Gasque,
Costamed,
Phone: 803-7777

UROLOGISTS

Dr. Jorge Carlos Aviles Rosado,
Centro Medico de las Americas
Calle 54 No. 365,
Por Av. Perez Ponce,
Col. Centro, Merida, Yuc.
Tel: 926-2745

Dr. Jorge Navarrete Fernandez,
Clinica de Merida,
Av. Itzaes No. 242.
Col. Garcia Gineres, Merida, Yuc.
Tel: 920-1986

HOSPITALS - PRIVATE

Centro Médico de las Américas
Address: Calle 54 #365
(at the corner of Avenida Pérez Ponce)
Colonia Centro, Mérida, Yuc.
Location: two blocks from U.S. Consulate
Main Phones: (999) 926-2111, 926-2619,
926-2732, 926-2354
Fax Phone: (999) 926-4710
Emergency Phone: (999) 927-3199
E-mail: cma@sureste.com
http://www.centromedicodelasamericas.com.mx/

Centro de Especialidades Medicas (CEM)
Calle 60 #329-B by 35 and Av. Colon
Col. Alcalá Martin
Phone: 920-4040
http://www.cemsureste.com/cem_index.htm
Emergencies: Ext. 111

Centro Medico Pensiones
Calle 7 #215-A
Col. Pensiones
Phone: 925-8019
http://centromedicopensiones.com/

Emergencies: Ext. 106

Clinica de Merida
Av. Itzaes No. 242
(between Calle 25 and Calle 27)
Colonia García Jineres, Mérida, Yuc.
Tel: (999) 942-1800, 920-0412, 920-0413,
920-0114
Emergencies: (999) 925-4508 ext 141,
925-3335
E-mail: clinmed@sureste.com
http://www.clinicademerida.com.mx/

Hospital Psiquiatrico Merida
Calle 116 no. 341, Por 59
Colonia Bojorques, Mérida, Yuc.n
Tel: (999) 945-1502

Hospital Star Medica
Calle 26 No. 199, Entre 15 y 7
Col. Altabrisa, Mérida, Yuc.
Tel: (999) 930-2880
http://www.starmedica.com/_ES/

Hospital Santelena
Calle 14 #81, by 5 and 7,
Col. San Antonio Cinta
Phone: 943-1333
Emergencies: Ext. 135

HOSPITALS - PUBLIC

Cruz Roja Mexicana
Av Quetzacoalt #104
Col. Centro
Phone: 983- 0233

Centro de Salud Publica
Calle 72 #463 Col. Centro
Phone: 928-6185

Clinica Materno-Infantil Maria Jose
Calle 53 Nº 484 by 54 & 56
Col. Centro
Phone: 928 5325
Dr. Sergio Manuel Perez Cervera

Hospital General O'Horan

Av. Itzaes, Por Av. Jacinto Canec
Mérida, Yuc.
Tel: (999) 930-3320
Fax: (999) 928-5507

Hospital Juarez
Av. Colón by Av. Itzaes,
Col. García Gineres, Mérida, Yuc.
Phone: 925-0831, 925-0866 ext. 2553

IMSS (Instituto Mexicano de Seguro Social, or
Mexican Institute of Social Security):
H. G. P. Torre de Especialidades
Calle 34 by 41 No. 439,
Ex-Terrenos El Fénix,
Col. Industrial, Mérida, Yuc.
Phone: 922-56-0601, 922-5656 ext. 4102

MEXICALI

CARDIOLOGISTS

Dr. Salvador Corral Villegas
Ave. Reforma #1004
Zona Centro
CP 21200
salvadorcorralmd@hotmail.com
554-1520
U.S. Cell: 760-234-3122

Dr. José A. Medina
Avenida Reforma #949-3
Zona Centro
Tel/Fax: (686) 554-0972
Home: (686) 568-3927
Cel: 044-686-581-8801
e-mail: adrimed@telnor.net

GENERAL MEDICINE

Dr. Alfredo Gruel
Avenida Madero #1060
Tel: (686) 553-4015, ext. 226

Fax: (686) 553-5235
Cel: 044-686-113-2905
e-mail: drgruel@almater.com

GYNECOLOGISTS

Dr. Leonardo Garza
Avenida Madero #946
Tel: (686) 552-3487
Home: (686) 552-4118
Cel: 044-686-840-2073
E-mail: garzal@telnor.net

INTERNISTS

Dr. Mario Lomeli Eguia
Ave. Madero No. 988
Mexicali, Baja California
Tel: (686) 554-2282

Dr. José A. Medina
Avenida Reforma #949-3
Zona Centro
Tel/Fax: (686) 554-0972
Home: (686) 568-3927
Cel: 044-686-581-8801
e-mail: adrimed@telnor.net

OBSTETRICIANS

Dr. Leonardo Garza
Avenida Madero #946
Tel: (686) 552-3487
Home: (686) 552-4118
Cel: 044-686-840-2073
E-mail: garzal@telnor.net

ORTHOPEDICIANS / TRAUMATOLOGISTS

Dr. Humberto Torres
Avenida Madero #836 (corner of Calle "A")
Zona Centro
Tel: (686) 552-6310
Fax: (686) 553-4161

Cel: 044-686-946-8226
e-mail: drhumbertotorres@hotmail.com

PEDIATRICIANS

Dr. Cipriano Aguilar
Calle Lerdo #1010
Colonia Segunda
Tel: (686) 551-9525
Home: (686) 554-6782
Cel: 044-686-157-0585
e-mail: cipra52@hotmail.com

SURGEONS

Dr. Alberto Aceves D.
Avenida Madero #1119-2
Tel: (686) 552-8191
Fax: (686) 554-6661
Cel: 044-686-946-1696
E-mail: aaceves@hotmail.com

HOSPITALS

Hospital Almater
Avenida Madero #1060
Colonia Nueva
Tel: (686) 553-4015
Fax: (686) 553-5235
website: http://www.almaterhospital.com/

Hospital Mexico Americano
Calle Reforma No. 1000 y Calle B
Mexicali, Baja California
Tel. & Fax: (686) 552-2300

MEXICO CITY

AMBULANCES

Ambulancia Santaella
Parque Lira 57, Local 2
Colonia San Miguel de Chapultepec
México, D.F.
Tel: (55) 5277-7999 / 5516-2691 / 2447

CARDIOLOGISTS

Dr. David Bialoztozky
Hospital ABC Observatorio
Calle Sur 136 No. 116, Office 519
Colonia de las Américas, México D.F.
Tel: (55) 5272-2406 / 2582
Radio: (55) 5230-3030 clave 11376

Dr. Victor M. Diaz
Internal Medicine, Cardiology
Address: Calle Puente de Piedra #150,
Office C-723, Tower 2
Borough: Colonia Toriello Guerra
Work: (55) 5424-7200 ext. 4430
Fax: (55) 5528-7238
Home: (55) 5655-5329
Mobile: 044-55-2135-7876
Email: diazv@portalmedico.com.mx
Pager: (55) 5227-7979, PIN# 5277946

Dr. Ursulo Juárez
Internal Medicine, Cardiology
Hospital Angeles de Pedregal
Address: Calle Camino a Santa Teresa #1055,
Office 810
Borough: Colonia Héroes de Padierna
Work/Fax: (55) 5652-3316
Mobile: 044-55-5413-8248
Pager: (55) 5227-7979, PIN# 5286599
Email: ujuarez@medmail.com

Dr. Eugenio A Ruesga

Hospital ABC Observatorio
Torre Mackenzie, Office 401
Calle Sur 136 No. 116
Colonia de las Américas
México D.F.
Tel: (55) 5272-2526
Fax: (55) 5272-3698
Radio: (55) 5629-9800 clave 9912990

Dr. Efrain Waisser
Internal Medicine, Cardiology &
Interventional Cardiology
Hospital ABC
Address: Fuente de Pirámides #1, 2nd floor
Borough: Colonia Tecamachalco
Work: (55) 5294-7166
Fax: (55) 5294-9776
Pager: (55) 5629-9800, PIN# 8173
Email: swaisser@infosel.net.mx

DENTISTS

Dr. Carlos Cornish
Félix Berenguer 106 - 401
Lomas de Virreyes, México D.F.
Tel: (55) 5540-2948 / 2946
Cell: (55) 5404-5117
Fax: (55) 5540-7543

Dr. Juan Claudio Lemionet Abascal
Kelvin 10 - 602
Col. Anzures, México D.F.
Tel: (55) 5531-5022 / 5545-8321

Dr. Miguel Macedo Zesati
Skydoc Implant Center
Acueducto Río Hondo 28 - 302
Lomas de Virreyes, México D.F.
Tel: (55) 5540-1402/03
Website: http://www.skydoc.com.mx/
Emergency services 24/7

Dra. Karla Ontiveros
Molière 39 - 803
Col. Polanco, México D.F
Tel: (55) 5280-0115 / 5060
Fax: (55) 5280-4327

Dr. Samuel Rajunov
Specialist in Pediatric Dentistry
Prado Sur 480
Colonia Lomas de Chapultepec, México D.F.
Tel/Fax: (55) 5202-1238

EAR, NOSE & THROAT

Dr. Benjamín Macías Jiménez
Hegel 120, Office 503
Col. Polanco
México D.F.
Tel: (55) 5545-2839
Fax: (55) 5531-8089

ENDOCRINOLOGISTS

Dr. Francisco Manzano
Internal Medicine, Endocrinology
Hospital Angeles Lomas
Address: Vialidad de la Barranca, no street
number, Office 670
Borough: Colonia del Valle de las Palmas
Work: (55) 5246-9474, 5246-9476, ext. 239
Fax: (55) 5246-9475
Pager: (55) 2581-3399, PIN# 5529663622
Email: fmanzano@icabim.com

ENDOSCOPY

Dr. Carlos Mitrani
Gastroentrology, Endoscopy
Hospital Angeles Lomas
Address: Vialidad de la Barranca, no street
number, Office 430
Borough: Colonia Valle de Las Palmas
Work: (55) 5246-9694
Fax: (55) 5246-9695
Pager: (55) 5629-9800, PIN# 1718
Email: carlosmitrani@aol.com

Dr. Jacobo Vestel K.
Internal Medicine, Gastroenterology,
Endoscopy
Hospital ABC
Address: Calle Fuente de Pirámides #1,

2nd floor, Office 201
Borough: Colonia Lomas de Tecamachalco
Work: (55) 5294-7166
Fax: (55) 5294-9776
Pager: (55) 5629-9800 PIN# 16134

FERTILITY

Dr. Alberto Kably
Obstetrics & Gynecology, Fertility & Sterility
Hospital Angeles Lomas
Address: Vialidad de la Barranca,
no street number, Office 240
Borough: Colonia Valle de Las Palmas
Work: (55) 5246-9410, 5246-9412
Fax: (55) 5246-9411
Pager: (55) 5328-2828, PIN# 1067
Email: cepam@infosel.net.mx

Dr. Guillermo Rocha
Obstetrics & Gynecology, Fertility
Hospital ABC
Address: Calle "Sur 136" #201, Office 101
Borough: Colonia las Américas
Work: (55) 5272-2045
Fax: (55) 5272-3988
Pager: (55) 5328-2828, PIN# 1107
Email: guillermorochadelvalle@yahoo.com

GASTROENTEROLOGISTS

Dra. Christiane Coté
ABC Hospital
Torre de Consultorios 116, Office 201
Calle Sur 136
Col. Las Américas, México D.F.
Tel: (55) 5277-0770 / 5273-6615
Fax: (55) 5273-6549

Dr. Carlos Mitrani
Gastroentrology, Endoscopy
Hospital Angeles Lomas
Address: Vialidad de la Barranca,
no street number, Office 430
Borough: Colonia Valle de Las Palmas
Work: (55) 5246-9694

Fax: (55) 5246-9695
Pager: (55) 5629-9800, PIN# 1718
Email: carlosmitrani@aol.com

Dr. Jacobo Vestel K.
Internal Medicine, Gastroenterology,
Endoscopy
Hospital ABC
Address: Calle Fuente de Pirámides #1,
2nd floor, Office 201
Borough: Colonia Lomas de Tecamachalco
Work: (55) 5294-7166
Fax: (55) 5294-9776
Pager: (55) 5629-9800 PIN# 16134

GENERAL PHYSICIANS

Dr. Franklin Krajmalnik
Roqueta 250
Col. Lomas de Bezares, México D.F.
Tel: (55) 5531-2562 / 5203-2368
Cell: (55) 5509-7894

Dr. Diana Morales
Varsovia 57, Office 301
(between Londres y Praga)
Col. Juárez, México D.F.
Tel: (55) 5514-3667
Cell: (55) 2955-0352

GYNECOLOGISTS

Dr. Francisco J. Bernardez
Obstetrics & Gynecology
Hospital Español de Beneficiencia
Address: Torcuato Tasso #335, Office 701
Work: (55) 5531-4087
Fax: (55) 5531-5277
Mobile: 044-55-5412-9458
Pager: (55) 5629-9800, PIN# 9922384
Email: frann60@igo.com.mx

Dr. Alfonso Gutiérrez Najar
Hospital Ángeles del Pedregal
Camino a Sta. Teresa 1055, Office 1282
Col. Héroes de Padierna, México D.F.
Tel: (55) 5652-1111

Fax: (55) 5652-9349

Dr. Alberto Kably
Obstetrics & Gynecology, Fertility & Sterility
Hospital Angeles Lomas
Address: Vialidad de la Barranca,
no street number, Office 240
Borough: Colonia Valle de Las Palmas
Work: (55) 5246-9410, 5246-9412
Fax: (55) 5246-9411
Pager: (55) 5328-2828, PIN# 1067
Email: cepam@infosel.net.mx

Dr. Joseph Michel
ABC Hospital
Torre de Consultorios, Office 304
Calle Sur 136
Colonia Las Américas, México D.F.
Tel/Fax: (55) 5272-3621 / 2822
Cell: (55) 3030-8789
E-mail: drjosephmichel@prodigy.net.mx

Dr. Guillermo Rocha
Obstetrics & Gynecology, Fertility
Hospital ABC
Address: Calle "Sur 136" #201, Office 101
Borough: Colonia las Américas
Work: (55) 5272-2045
Fax: (55) 5272-3988
Pager: (55) 5328-2828, PIN# 1107
Email: guillermorochadelvalle@yahoo.com

IMMUNOLOGISTS

Dr. Arnoldo Kraus
Internal Medicine, Immunology, and
Rheumatology
Hospital ABC
Address: Calle "Sur 136" #116, Office 405
Borough: Colonia las Américas
Work: (55) 5272-2484
Fax: (55) 5272-2599
Home: (55) 5293-0850
Pager: (55) 5328-2828, PIN# 1231

INTERNISTS

Dr. Miguel Ahumada
Endocrinologist
Hospital Ángeles del Pedregal
Torre Ángeles, Office 842
Periférico Sur 3697
Col. Héroes de Padierna
México D.F.
Tel/Fax: (55) 5652-7776

Dr. Victor M. Diaz
Internal Medicine, Cardiology
Address: Calle Puente de Piedra #150,
Office C-723, Tower 2
Borough: Colonia Toriello Guerra
Work: (55) 5424-7200 ext. 4430
Fax: (55) 5528-7238
Home: (55) 5655-5329
Mobile: 044-55-2135-7876
Email: diazv@portalmedico.com.mx
Pager: (55) 5227-7979, PIN# 5277946

Dr. Luis Guevara
Internal Medicine, Nephrology
Hospital Médica Sur
Address: Calle Puente de Piedra #150
Borough: Colonia Toriello Guerra
Work/Fax: (55) 5424-7200 ext. 4429
Pager: (55) 5230-3030, PIN# 19751
Email: lga2k@yahoo.com

Dr. Arnoldo Kraus
Internal Medicine, Immunology, and
Rheumatology
Hospital ABC
Address: Calle "Sur 136" #116, Office 405
Borough: Colonia las Américas
Work: (55) 5272-2484
Fax: (55) 5272-2599
Home: (55) 5293-0850
Pager: (55) 5328-2828, PIN# 1231

Dr. Ursulo Juárez
Internal Medicine, Cardiology
Hospital Angeles de Pedregal
Address: Calle Camino a Santa Teresa #1055,
Office 810

Borough: Colonia Héroes de Padierna
Work/Fax: (55) 5652-3316
Mobile: 044-55-5413-8248
Pager: (55) 5227-7979, PIN# 5286599
Email: ujuarez@medmail.com

Dr. Francisco Manzano
Internal Medicine, Endocrinology
Hospital Angeles Lomas
Address: Vialidad de la Barranca,
no street number, Office 670
Borough: Colonia del Valle de las Palmas
Work: (55) 5246-9474, 5246-9476, ext. 239
Fax: (55) 5246-9475
Pager: (55) 2581-3399, PIN# 5529663622
Email: fmanzano@icabim.com

Dra. Aurora Orzechowski
Internal Medicine
Hospital Angeles Pedregal
Address: Periférico Sur #3697, Office 650
Borough: Colonia Héroes de Padierna
Work: (55) 5568-6859, 5568-5500, ext. 111
Fax: (55) 5135-4748
Mobile: 044-55-5503-3749
Pager: (55) 5227-7979, PIN# 5254754
Email: orche19@prodigy.net.mx

Dr. Ildefonso Téllez
Internal Medicine, Infectious Diseases
Hospital Angeles Lomas
Address: Vialidad de la Barranca,
no street number, Office 430
Borough: Colonia Valle de las Palmas
Work: (55) 5246-9694, 5246-9695
Fax: (55) 5246-9696
Mobile: 044-55-1921-2727
Pager: (55) 5629-9800, PIN# 9963006
Email: ilteg@hotmail.com

Dr. Jesús J. Vázquez C.
Internal Medicine, Pulmonology
Hospital Angeles Lomas
Address: Vialidad de la Barranca,
no street number, Office 430
Borough: Colonia Valle de las Palmas
Work: (55) 5246-9696, 5246-9697
Fax: (55) 5246-9694

Home: (55) 5343-3369
Mobile: 044-55-5500-9125
Pager: (55) 5629-9800, PIN# 9937045
Email: lungdoc@terra.com.mx

Dr. Jacobo Vestel K.
Internal Medicine, Gastroenterology,
Endoscopy
Hospital ABC
Address: Calle Fuente de Pirámides #1,
2nd floor, Office 201
Borough: Colonia Lomas de Tecamachalco
Work: (55) 5294-7166
Fax: (55) 5294-9776
Pager: (55) 5629-9800 PIN# 16134

Dr. Efrain Waisser
Internal Medicine, Cardiology &
Interventional Cardiology
Hospital ABC
Address: Fuente de Pirámides #1, 2nd floor
Borough: Colonia Tecamachalco
Work: (55) 5294-7166
Fax: (55) 5294-9776
Pager: (55) 5629-9800, PIN# 8173
Email: swaisser@infosel.net.mx

LABORATORIES

Laboratorios Quest Diagnostics Polanco
Edgar Allan Poe 108
Col. Polanco, México DF
Tel: (55) 5281-7802
Hours: Monday to Friday, 7-16
Saturday, 7:30-13:30

LAPARASCOPIC SURGERY

Dr. Denzil E. Garteiz
General and Laparoscopic Surgery
Hospital Angeles Lomas
Address: Vialidad de la Barranca,
no street number, Office 410
Borough: Colonia Valle de Las Palmas
Work: (55) 5246-9527
Mobile: 044-55-1089-6635

Pager: (55) 5278-4848, PIN# 5510896635
Email: denzilgarteiz@yahoo.com

NEPHROLOGISTS

Dr. Luis Guevara
Internal Medicine, Nephrology
Hospital Médica Sur
Address: Calle Puente de Piedra #150
Borough: Colonia Toriello Guerra
Work/Fax: (55) 5424-7200 ext. 4429
Pager: (55) 5230-3030, PIN# 19751
Email: lga2k@yahoo.com

OBSTETRICIANS

Dr. Francisco J. Bernardez
Obstetrics & Gynecology
Hospital Español de Beneficiencia
Address: Torcuato Tasso #335, Office 701
Work: (55) 5531-4087
Fax: (55) 5531-5277
Mobile: 044-55-5412-9458
Pager: (55) 5629-9800, PIN# 9922384
Email: frann60@igo.com.mx

Dr. Alfonso Gutiérrez Najar
Hospital Ángeles del Pedregal
Camino a Sta. Teresa 1055, Office 1282
Col. Héroes de Padierna
México D.F.
Tel: (55) 5652-1111
Fax: (55) 5652-9349

Dr. Joseph Michel
ABC Hospital
Torre de Consultorios, Office 304
Calle Sur 136
Colonia Las Américas, México D.F.
Tel/Fax: (55) 5272-3621 / 2822
Cell: (55) 3030-8789
E-mail: drjosephmichel@prodigy.net.mx
Hours: Monday-Friday, 10-16

Dr. Alberto Kably
Obstetrics & Gynecology, Fertility & Sterility
Hospital Angeles Lomas

Address: Vialidad de la Barranca,
no street number, Office 240
Borough: Colonia Valle de Las Palmas
Work: (55) 5246-9410, 5246-9412
Fax: (55) 5246-9411
Pager: (55) 5328-2828, PIN# 1067
Email: cepam@infosel.net.mx

Dr. Guillermo Rocha
Obstetrics & Gynecology, Fertility
Hospital ABC
Address: Calle "Sur 136" #201, Office 101
Borough: Colonia las Américas
Work: (55) 5272-2045
Fax: (55) 5272-3988
Pager: (55) 5328-2828, PIN# 1107
Email: guillermorochadelvalle@yahoo.com

OPHTALMOLOGISTS

Dr. Nathan Grinberg
Hegel 120, office 602
Col. Polanco, México D.F.
Tel: (55) 5250-0268
Emergencies: (55) 1320-8074
Fax: (55) 5531-3730

Dr. David Lozano Elizondo
Patriotismo 880
Col. Insurgentes - Mixcoac, México D.F.
Tel: (55) 5563-8042
Fax: (55) 5615-7375

Dr. Benjamín Zagorín
Paseo de las Palmas 745, office 101
Col. Lomas de Chapultepec
México D.F.
Tel and Fax: (55) 5540-1243 / 5520-3693

ORTHOPEDISTS / PHYSIOTHERAPISTS

Dr. Luis Castañeda
Hospital ABC Santa Fe
Av. Carlos Graes Fernández 154, Office 405
Col. Tlaxala, México D.F.

Tel: (55) 1664-7064
Fax: (55) 1664-7161
Emergencies: (55) 5629-9800 clave 876
2nd office:
Sierra Nevada 234
Col. Lomas de Chapultepec, México D.F.
Tel/Fax: (55) 5540-7740, 5202-4176 / 3960

Dr. José Antonio Velutini
Orthopedics/Traumatology
Hospital ABC
Address: Calle "Sur 136" #116, Office 411
Borough: Colonia las Américas
Work: (55) 5272-3765
Pager: (55) 5629-9800, PIN# 17783
Email: drjavelutini@yahoo.com.mx

PEDIATRICIANS

Dr. Eduardo Emilio Carsi Bocanegra
Hospital Ángeles del Pedregal
Torre Ángeles, Office 740
Camino a Santa Teresa 1055
Col. Héroes de Padierna
México D.F.
Tel: (55) 5652-7042 / 62
Fax: (55) 5568-5888

Dr. Agustin de Colsa R.
Pediatrics and Infectious Diseases
Hospital Angeles Lomas
Address: Vialidad de la Barranca,
no street number, Office 360
Borough: Colonia Valle de Las Palmas
Work: (55) 5246-9400
Mobile: 044-55-5455-5414
Email: adcdoe@yahoo.com

Dr. Sergio Graham P.
Neonatologist
Hospital Ángeles del Pedregal
Torre de Especialidades Quirúrgicas,
Office 1082 A
Camino a Santa Teresa 1055
Col. Héroes de Padierna, México DF
Tel and Fax: (55) 5652-2011 ext. 4082
Work: (55) 5652-5225, 5652-7280

Fax: (55) 5652-5225
Email: graham@ragnatela.net.mx,
scotland@avantel.net

Dr. José A. Hernández
Pediatrics, Neonatology
Hospital Medica Sur
Address: Calle Puente de Piedra #150,
Tower 2, Office 310
Borough: Colonia Toriello Guerra
Work: (55) 5606-7159, 5424-7200, ext. 2217
Pager: (55) 5227-7979, PIN# 5262067
Email: jhernandez@medicasur.org.mx

Dr. Roberto Hirsch
Grupo Médico Pediátrico
Prado Sur 290
México D.F.
Tel: (55) 1100-1200 press #0

Dr. David Nobigrot Kleinman
Neonatologist
Benjamin Hill 217
between Saltillo and Ometusco
Col. Condesa,México D.F.
Tel: (55) 5272-7175/5516-7300

2nd office:
José Luis Lagrange 225
between Homero and Horacio
Col. Polanco, México D.F.
Tel: (55) 5557-8639
Emergencies:
Pager: (55) 5629-9800 code: 46944
Cell: (55) 5506-4449

Dr. Alberto Orozco
Pediatrics, Neonatology
Hosptial Angeles de Pedregal
Address: Periférico Sur #3697, Office 620
Borough: Colonia Héroes de Padierna
Work: (55) 5568-4091
Fax: (55) 5652-8688
Mobile: 044-55-5431-2255
Pager: (55) 5629-9800, PIN# 16152
Email: orozco@netmex.com.mx

PSYCHOLOGISTS

Psic. Sharon Blanco Vega
Tabasco 56 corner with Frontera
Colonia Roma, México D.F.
Tel: (55) 2454-3329
Cell: (55) 1343-2445
E-mail: ibizabaleares@hotmail.com;
prevea@hotmail.com

PULMONOLOGISTS

Dr. Jesús J. Vázquez C.
Internal Medicine, Pulmonology
Hospital Angeles Lomas
Address: Vialidad de la Barranca,
no street number, Office 430
Borough: Colonia Valle de las Palmas
Work: (55) 5246-9696, 5246-9697
Fax: (55) 5246-9694
Home: (55) 5343-3369
Mobile: 044-55-5500-9125
Pager: (55) 5629-9800, PIN# 9937045
Email: lungdoc@terra.com.mx

REUMATHOLOGISTS

Dr. Arnoldo Kraus
Internal Medicine, Immunology, and
Rheumatology
Hospital ABC
Address: Calle "Sur 136" #116, Office 405
Borough: Colonia las Américas
Work: (55) 5272-2484
Fax: (55) 5272-2599
Home: (55) 5293-0850
Pager: (55) 5328-2828, PIN# 1231

FERTILITY

Dr. Alberto Kably
Obstetrics & Gynecology, Fertility & Sterility
Hospital Angeles Lomas
Address: Vialidad de la Barranca,
no street number, Office 240

Borough: Colonia Valle de Las Palmas
Work: (55) 5246-9410, 5246-9412
Fax: (55) 5246-9411
Pager: (55) 5328-2828, PIN# 1067
Email: cepam@infosel.net.mx

SURGEONS

Dr. Jorge Cervantes
General Surgeon
Hospital ABC
Address: Calle "Sur 136" #116, Office 508
Borough: Colonia las Américas
Work: (55) 5272-3410, 5272-2244,
5596-0730
Fax: (55) 5516-9970
Home: (55) 5596-0730
Mobile: 044-55-5500-0909
Pager: (55) 5230-3030, PIN# Alfa2
Email: jcervantes@abchospital.com

Dr. Denzil E. Garteiz
General and Laparoscopic Surgery
Hospital Angeles Lomas
Address: Vialidad de la Barranca,
no street number, Office 410
Borough: Colonia Valle de Las Palmas
Work: (55) 5246-9527
Mobile: 044-55-1089-6635
Pager: (55) 5278-4848, PIN# 5510896635
Email: denzilgarteiz@yahoo.com

Dr. Salvador Medina
Hospital Ángeles del Pedregal
Camino a Santa Teresa 1055, Office 503
Col. Héroes de Padierna, México D.F.
Tel: (55) 5568-5083
Fax: (55) 5652-1906

Dr. Gonzálo Torres
Hospital Ángeles del Pedregal
Torre Ángeles, Office 625
Camino a Santa Teresa 1055
Col. Héroes de Padierna
México D.F.
Tel and Fax: (55) 5652-2271

TRAUMATOLOGY

Dr. José Antonio Velutini
Orthopedics/Traumatology
Hospital ABC
Address: Calle "Sur 136" #116, Office 411
Borough: Colonia las Américas
Work: (55) 5272-3765
Pager: (55) 5629-9800, PIN# 17783
Email: drjavelutini@yahoo.com.mx

UROLOGIST

Dr. Leopoldo García Bravo
Hospital Ángeles del Pedregal
Torre Ángeles, Office 822
Camino a Santa Teresa 1055
Colonia Héroes de Padierna
México D.F.
Tel: (55) 5135-2749 / 5652-3011 ext. 4822/23
Fax: (55) 5135-2749

VETERINARIANS

Dr. Carlos García
Miguel de Cervantes Saavedra 625
Colonia Irrigación, México D.F.
Tel: (55) 5557-0875 & 2619

CLINICS (SPANISH ONLY)

Clinica Guerrero
Calle Guerrero 107
Colonia Guerrero, México, D.F.
Tel: (55) 5546-3249

Clinica Portales
Municipio Libre 97
(near Metro Portales)
Colonia Portales, México, D.F.
Tel: (55) 5539-5320

Clinica Tacubaya
Av. Revolución 309
(between Héroes de Padierna y Tacubaya)
Colonia Tacubaya, México, D.F.
Tel: (55) 5516-7072

Cruz Roja (Red Cross)
Ejército Nacional 1032
Colonia Polanco, México, D.F.
Tel: 5395-1111 (operator) ext. 173
Emergencies: 065

Medica Movil / Unidad Movil de
Terapia Intensiva
Porfirio Díaz 66
Colonia Noche Buena, México, D.F.
Tel: (55) 5598-6222 / 5582-3700

HOSPITALS

American British Cowdray (ABC) Hospital
Address: Calle "Sur 136" #116
Borough: Colonia Las Américas
Second location in Santa Fe: Avenida Carlos
Graef Fernandez 154, Col. Tlaxala
Santa Fe, Cuajimalpa, DF
Main Phone #: (55) 5230-8000, 5230-8080
Fax Phone #: (55) 5230-8028, 5230-8146
Emergency Phone #: (55) 5230-8161,
5230-8162, 5230-8163, 5230-8164

Beneficencia Español (Hospital Español)
Ejército Nacional 613
Colonia Granada, México D.F.
Tel: (55) 5255-9600
Emergencies: (55) 5255-9645
Fax: (55) 5255-9665
(Spanish only)

Centro Médico
Dalinde Tuxpan 25 y Baja California
Col. Roma Sur
5265-28-00 5265-28-05

Clinica Londres
Durango No. 50,
Col. Roma
5229-84-00

Clinica Sinaloa
Arquitectos 21 Interior 2
Col. Escandón, México, D. F.
5256-2997 5273-9428 04455-2758-8367

Hospital ABC
Calle Sur 136 No. 116
Esq. Observatorio
Col. Las Américas, México, D.F.
Tel: (55) 5230-8000 (dial 1 for emergencies)
Fax: (55) 5230-8146

Hospital Angeles del Pedregal
Camino a Santa Teresa No. 1055
Col. Heroes de Padierna
5652-30-11 5652-20-11

Hospital Angeles Mocel
Gelati 29
Col. San Miguel Chapultepec, México, D.F.
Tel: (55) 5278-2300 / 2600 (dial 7 for
emergencies)
Emergencies: (55) 5277-3020
Fax: (55) 5273-7720
(Spanish)

Hospital Angeles-Lomas
Address: Avenida Vialidad de la Barranca,
no street number
Borough: Colonia Valle de las Palmas
Notable Landmarks: Center of InterLomas
Main Phone: (55) 5246-5000, ext.
5332, 5347
Fax Phone: (55) 5246-5218
Emergency Phone #: (55) 5246-5096,
5246-5097

Hospital Angeles de Pedregal
Address: Calle Camino Santa Teresa #1055
Borough: Colonia Héroes de Padierna
Main Phone: (55) 5449-5500
Fax Phone: (55) 5652-8598
Emergency Phone: (55) 5568-1540,
5652-6987

Hospital Balbuena
Calzada Cecilio Robelo 103
Corner with Calle Sur
Col. Aeronáutica Militar
México, D.F.
Tel: (55) 5764-3053 (emergencies) /
5764-3054 (Switchboard)
(Spanish)

Hospital de Enfermedades Respiratorias
Calzada de Tlalpan 4502
Seccion 16, Tlalpan, D.F.
5666-45-39

Hospital de Especialidades Belisario
Dominguez
Ave. Tláhuac 4866
Corner with Zacatlán de las Manzanas
Col. San Lorenzo Tezonco, México, D.F.
Tel: (55) 5850-0000 / 20
Ext. 1032 (emergencies)

Hospital Médica Sur
Address: Calle Puente de Piedra #150
Borough: Colonia Toriello Guerra, Tlalpan
Main Phone #: (55) 5424-7200
Fax Phone #: (55) 5606-1651
Emergency Phone #: (55) 5666-7059

Hospital de la Mujer Prolongacion Salvador
Diaz Miron 374 Col. Santo Tomas
Close to Subway Station
Colegio Militar
5341-1100

Hospital de Mexico
Agrarismo 208,
Col. Escandon
5516-99-00 al 19

Hospital Español
Av. Ejercito Nacional No. 613
Col. Granada
4959-6100

Hospital General Balbuena (DDF)
Cecilio Robelo y Sur # 103
Col. Aeronautica Militar
5552-1602,05 5764-0157 5552-66-68
5764-30-53 5552-16-07
Emergency 5552-00-05

Hospital General Ticoman
Plan de San Luis (no street number)
Col. Ticoman
5754-30-12 5754-33-44 5754-39-39

Hospital Infantil de Mexico
Dr. Marquez # 162
Col. Doctores
5761-01-03

Hospital Infantil Privado
Viaducto Rio Becerra
No. 97 Col. Napoles
5682-50-00 5687-30-55 5340-10-00

Hospital Juarez
Av. Politecnico No. 5160
Col. Magadalena de las Salinas
2973-2229 5747-7560
Emergency Ext. 471

Hospital La Villa
Ave. San Juan de Aragón 285
Col. Granjas Modernas, México, D.F.
Tel: (55) 5750-3012
(Spanish)

Hospital Metropolitano
Tlacotalpan No. 59
Col. Roma Sur
5265-18-00 5265-19-00

Hospital Mocel
Gelati No. 29
Col. San Miguel Chapultepec
5278-23-00

Hospital Pediatrico Coyoacan
Moctezuma # 18
Col. El Carmen
5554-28-58 to 62

Hospital Pediatrico Peralvillo
Tolnahuac No. 14
Col. San Simon Tolnahuac
Del. Cuauhtemoc, Mexico, D. F.
Director Gral. Dr. Hector Sucilla
5583-38-12 5583-38-01 5583-38-23
5583-39-48 5583-41-80

Hospital Peralvillo
Tolnahuac # 14
Col. San Simon Tolnahuac
5583-41-80 5583-38-23 5583-38-01

Hospital Ruben Lenero
Plan de San Luis y Diaz Miron
Col. Santo Tomas
Cerca Hospital de la Mujer
5341-45-80 5341-26-55

Hospital Star Medica Infantil Privado
Viaducto Río Becerra 97
Col. Nápoles, México, D.F.
Tel: (55) 5340-1000 press 1 for emergencies
Fax: (55) 5669-0404
(Spanish)

Hospital Tacubaya
Carlos Lazo# 25 corner of Gaviota
Col. Tacubaya
5515-61-70

Hospital Xoco
Ave. México Coyoacán (no street number)
Corner with Calle Bruno Traven
Col. General Anaya, México, D.F.
Tel: (55) 5688-9015 /9115 (emergencies)
(Spanish)

Instituto de Nutricion Salvador Zubiran
Vasco de Quiroga # 15
Col. Seccion 16, Tlalpan
5487-0900

IInstituto Nacional de Cardiologia
(Heart Attacks)
Juan Badiano 1
Esq. Periférico Sur y Viaducto
Colonia Sección 16 Del. Tlalpan, México, D.F.
Tel: (55) 5573-2911 / 5255
Emergencies: extension 333 or 1260
Fax: (55) 5573-0994
(Spanish)

Instituto Nacional de Pediatria
Dr. Rogelio Paredes, Director of Hematology
Insurgentes Sur 3700-c
Close to Perisur Mall
Mexico, D.F.
5606-00-02

Instituto Para la Atencion del Nino Quemado
Prolongacion 16 de Septiembre Esq.
Camino a Nativitas
Col. Xaltogan Del. Xochimilco
5676-49-93

Medica Sur
Puente de Piedra 150
Col. Toriello Guerra Tlalpan, D.F.
5606-60-11 5606-22-77 5606-62-22
5424-72-73

Sanatorio Durango
Durango 296,
Col. Roma
5148-46-46

Shriners' Hospital
Calle Suchil No. 152
5618-47-50 5618-11-20 5618-49-85

PSYCHIATRIC HOSPITALS

Clinica Florida (Private clinic)
Ixtlacíhuatl 180
Col. Florida, México, D.F.
Tel: (55) 5661-0491 / 3371 / 5661
Fax: (55) 5663-5580
(Spanish)

Clinica San Rafael
Insurgentes Sur No. 4177
Col. Santa Ursula Xitla
5655-47-99 5573-42-66 5655-47-04

Hospital Psiquiatrico Fray Bernardino
Alvarez Av. Niño Jesús 2
Esq. San Buenaventura
Delegación Tlalpan
México, D.F.
Tel: (55) 5573-1500 / 1550
Fax: (55) 5573-0388
(Spanish)

BLOOD BANK

National Blood Transfusion Centre
Othón de Mendizábal 195
Col. Zacatenco, México, D.F.
Tel: (55) 5119-4620 to 28
To donate: 01-800-366-2636

MONTERREY

AMBULANCES

7/24 Asistencia Medica Inmediata
Belisario Dominguez 2005
Col. Obispado, Monterrey
Tel: (81) 8174-3501
Emergencies: (81) 8372-4724

Promedic
2 de Abril 706
Col. Independencia, Monterrey
Tel: (81) 8114-8877
Fax: (81) 8114-8811

CARDIOLOGISTS

Dr. Mario Benavides
Ecuador 2331, Office 837
Col. Balcones de Galerías, Monterrey
Tel: (81) 8347-4177 / 8347-5177
Emergencies: (81) 8380-4500 Clave 18896
E-mail: cecim.benavides@gmail.com

Dr. Héctor Fernández González
Autonomous University of Nuevo León, 1955
Instituto de Cardiología del Tecnológico
Centro Médico Zambrano Hellion del ITESM
Office (81) 8888-0500
Home (81) 8356-8485
Cellular 044-811-050-5781

Dr. Enrique Ponce de León
Internal Medicine, Cardiology
Address: Avenida Hidalgo #2030
Poniente (between Cerro de Picachos
and Boudelier streets)
Borough: Colonia Obispado
Work: (81) 8333-3366
Pager: (81) 8151-1111, PIN# 5120262
Mobile: 044-81-1475-2871
Email: eponcem@intercable.net

DENTISTS

Dr. Mario Chapa
Doctor Vera 100
Col. Los Doctores, Monterrey
Tel: (81) 8347-3223 / 8346-7030
E-mail: mariochapa@doctor.com

Dr. Juan Fidalgo Cavazos
Specializing In: General Dentistry
Pedodontist (Children's Dentist)
Autonomous University of Nuevo León, 1959
Loma Alta # 329 on the corner of
Loma Jardín,
Col. Loma Larga, Monterrey
Office Hours: 15 - 18:30
Office (81) 8342-9928
Home (81) 8345-3145
Email hildafidalgo@hotmail.com

Dr. Alejandro Muraira Flores
Specializing In: General Dentistry,
Pedodontist & Children's Dentist
Autonomous University of Nuevo León,
1983 Centro Médico Obispado
Hidalgo # 2530 Poniente, Room 313,
Col. Obispado, Monterrey
Office (81) 8333-8756
Home (81) 8333-9946
Cellular 044-811-240-6279
Email alejandromuraira@gmail.com

Dr. Serapio Manuel Muraira Garza
Specializing In: General Dentistry
Autonomous University of Nuevo León,
1956 Centro Médico Obispado
Hidalgo #2530 Poniente, Room 312,
Col. Obispado, Monterrey
Office (81) 8346-8091

DERMATOLOGISTS

Dra. Aida Grunspan
Loma Grande 2717, Mezzanine 11
Col. Loma de San Francisco, Monterrey, N.L.
Tel: (81) 8143-0560 / 1644-1668
E-mail: agrunspan@yahoo.com

Dr. Oliverio Welsh Lozano
Autonomous University of Nuevo León
Centro de Especialidades Médicas
J. Benítez # 2704,
Col. Obispado, Monterrey
Office (81) 8333-1466 & 8333-0107
Fax (81) 8333-2993
Home (81) 8338-4900 & 8338-4514

EAR, NOSE & THROAT

Dr. Alejandro Camelo Schwarz
Autonomous University of Nuevo León
Rio San Juan # 103, 2nd Floor,
Col. Miravalle, Monterrey
Office (81) 8356-7244 & 8356-8213
Email alejnadrocamelo@prodigy.net.mx

Dr. Jesús Jiménez Guzmán
Specializing In: Ear, Nose, Throat
Autonomous University of Nuevo León, 1959
Language: Spanish
Centro Médico Origen
Ruperto Martínez # 1321 Poniente,
entre Vallarta y Porfirio Díaz,
Col. Centro, Monterrey,
Office (81) 8343-2276 & 8343-2367
Email jesusjimenezg@hotmail.com

Dr. José de Jesús Rodríguez Martínez
Hidalgo # 2601 Poniente,
Col. Jardín Del Obispado, Monterrey
Office (81) 8346-2228, 8333-2345
Fax (81) 8346-8253
Email drjesusrodriguez@yahoo.com.mx

Dr. Carlos Salinas
Autonomous University of Nuevo León
Centro Médico Obispado
Hidalgo # 2625, entre Andes y
Privada Muguerza,
Col. Jardín Obispado, Monterrey
Office (81) 8346-6130
Cell Phone 044-811-660-1927
Email dr.salinas.orl@gmail.com

ENDOCRINOLOGISTS

Dr. Sergio Zuñiga
Doctors Hospital
Ecuador 2331, Office 837
Col. Balcones de Galerías, Monterrey
Tel. (81) 1365-8738 / 39
E-mail: sergiozungua@gmail.com

GASTROENTEROLOGISTS

Dr. Luis A. Morales
Internal Medicine, Gastroenterology
Address: Avenida Morones Prieto #3000
Poniente, Office 306
Borough: Colonia Los Doctores
Work: (81) 8333-2068, 8348-1447
Fax: (81) 8347-4833
Mobile: 044-81-8063-8432
Pager: (81) 8151-1111, PIN# 57411
Email: lumorale@itesm.mx

Dr. Leonel Rodríguez Reyna
Autonomous University of Nuevo León, 1965
Centro de Diagnóstico de Monterrey
Dr. Cantú # 300,
Col. Los Doctores, Monterrey
Office (81) 8346-9000 ext 131
& 8333-1450

GENERAL SURGEONS

Dr. Jorge E. Balli
General Surgery, Basic/Advanced Laparoscopy
Address: Calle Dr. Cantú #300, 6th floor
Borough: Colonia Los Doctores
Work: (81) 8333-6666
Fax: (81) 8333-6699
Mobile: 044-81-1212-0257
Pager: (81) 8151-1111, PIN# 516070
Email: jballi@hsj.com.mx

Dr. Jorge M. Garza Tijerina
Specializing In: General Surgery
Autonomous University of Nuevo León, 1963
Centro Médico Metropolitano

Av. Del Hospital # 110, Room 201,
Col. Sertoma, Monterrey
Office Hours: 10-1 & 4-7
Office (81) 8348-8695
Home (81) 8356-2465

Dr. Ignacio Javier Guzmán Valdez
Specializing In: General Surgery, Vascular
Surgery
Autonomous University of Nuevo León,
1972, FACS Minnesota University
Centro Médico Muguerza
Hidalgo Poniente # 2527, Room 305,
Col. Obispado, Monterrey
Office (81) 8333-0838, 8882-9238
Home (81) 8303-3648
Email driguzman@hotmail.com

Dr. Francisco X. Treviño
General Surgery, Laproscopic Surgery
Address: Avenida Morones Prieto #3000
Poniente, Office #8
Borough: Colonia Los Doctores
Work: (81) 8143-0330, 8143-0440
Fax: (81) 8347-0500
Home: (81) 8378-5557
Mobiles: 044-81-8324-3355,
044-81-8063-7412
Email: fxtrevino@hotmail.com,
franciscot@hsj.com.mx
Pager: (81) 8151-1111, PIN# 56077

GYNECOLOGISTS

Dr. Justo Cárdenas
Specializing In: Gynecology and Obstetrics
Autonomous University of Nuevo León,
1950 Centro Profesional Delta
Av. La Clínica # 2520, 4th Floor, Room 409,
Col. Sertoma, Monterrey
Office (81) 8346-2222
Home (81) 8356-8086

Dr. Carlos Félix
Obstetrics & Gynecology
Address: Calle "Dr. Cantú" #300, 5th floor
Borough: Colonia Los Doctores

Work/Fax: (81) 8333-3323
Home: (81) 8336-5404
Mobile: 044-81-8362-7036
Pager: (81) 8151-1111, PIN# 56598
Email: carfelar@infosel.net.mx

Dr. Heriberto Reyes Vidales
Specializing In: Gynecology and Obstetrics
Autonomous University of Nuevo León,
1969 Centro Médico Conchita
15 De Mayo # 1822 Poniente, 4th Floor,
Room 402,
Col. Centro, Monterrey
Office (81) 8347-0256
Home (81) 8315-2826
Cellular 044-818-162-2501
Email drheribertorv@prodigy.net.mx

INTENSIVE CARE

Dr. Felipe Pérez-Rada
Internal Medicine, Intensive Care
Address: Avenida La Clínica #2520, Office 525
Borough: Colonia Sertoma
Work: (81) 8348-9729
Mobile: 044-81-8309-3062
Pager: (81) 8380-4500, PIN# 3578
Email: fperez@hsj.com.mx

INTERNISTS

Dr. Bonifacio Aguilar
Specializing In: Internal Medicine (Internist &
Rheumatologist)
Autonomous University of Nuevo León, 1954
Centro de Especialidades Médicas
J. Benítez # 2704, 2nd Floor, Room 209,
Col. Obispado, Monterrey, Nuevo León,
Office Hours 9:30-11:30 & 2-6:20
Office (81) 8333-1466 & 8220-4444
Home (81) 8322-0444
Fax (81) 8333-2993

Dr. José Fernando Castilleja
Specializing In: Internal Medicine and
Critical care
Hospital San José
Avenida I. Morones Prieto # 3000 Poniente,
Col. Los Doctores, Monterrey,
Office (81) 1133-4400, 8040-6193
Office (81) 8347-1010 ext. 6193
Nextel (81) 1113-1761
Cellular 044-811-609-4119
Email fcastilleja@itesm.mx

Dr. Mario César González
Specializing In: Cardiology, Internal Medicine
Autonomous University of Nuevo León,
1961 Centro Profesional Delta
Av. La Clínica # 2520, Rooms 205 & 207,
Col. Sertomaj, Monterrey
Office Hours: 9:30-12 & 3:30-6
Office (81) 8348-8811 & 8348-7495
Home (81) 8356-3022 & 8378-1673
Cellular 044-818-362-7301

Dr. Luis A. Morales
Internal Medicine, Gastroenterology
Address: Avenida Morones Prieto #3000
Poniente, Office 306
Borough: Colonia Los Doctores
Work: (81) 8333-2068, 8348-1447
Fax: (81) 8347-4833
Mobile: 044-81-8063-8432
Pager: (81) 8151-1111, PIN# 57411
Email: lumorale@itesm.mx

Dr. Felipe Pérez-Rada
Internal Medicine, Intensive Care
Address: Avenida La Clínica #2520,
Office 525
Borough: Colonia Sertoma
Work: (81) 8348-9729
Mobile: 044-81-8309-3062
Pager: (81) 8380-4500, PIN# 3578
Email: fperez@hsj.com.mx

Dr. Enrique Ponce de León
Internal Medicine, Cardiology
Address: Avenida Hidalgo #2030 Poniente
(between Cerro de Picachos
and Boudelier streets)
Borough: Colonia Obispado
Work: (81) 8333-3366
Pager: (81) 8151-1111, PIN# 5120262
Mobile: 044-81-1475-2871
Email: eponcem@intercable.net

Dr. Roberto Rodriguez
Centro Médico Hidalgo
Ave. Hidalgo 1842 Pte.
Col. Obispado, Monterrey
Tel: (81) 8318-6949

Dr. Jorge Villarreal
Specializing In: Internal Medicine,
Cardiology
Autonomous University of Nuevo León,
1956 Centro Médico Hidalgo
Hidalgo # 2425 Poniente, 9th Floor,
Rooms 906 & 908,
Col. Obispado, Monterrey
Office Hours: 9-12 & 3-7
Office (81) 8318-6744 / 45
Fax (81) 8318-6798
Home (81) 8378-2966 & 8356-1277
Cellular 044-818-280-1978

LAPAROSCOPIC SURGEONS

Dr. Jorge E. Balli
General Surgery, Basic/Advanced
Laparoscopy
Address: Calle Dr. Cantú #300, 6th floor
Borough: Colonia Los Doctores
Work: (81) 8333-6666
Fax: (81) 8333-6699
Mobile: 044-81-1212-0257
Pager: (81) 8151-1111, PIN# 516070
Email: jballi@hsj.com.mx

Dr. José Fernando De la Garza
Specializing In: Orthopedics,
Traumatologist, Microsurgery
Autonomous University of Nuevo León,
1977 Centro Medico San José
Av. I. Morones Prieto # 3000, 7th Floor,
Col. Los Doctores, Monterrey
Office (81) 8333-2033, 8333-2333
Fax (81) 8333-3396
Mobile: 044-81-8185-3322
Pager: (81) 8151-1111, PIN# 18077
Email: jfdelag@hsj.com.mx

Dr. Francisco X. Treviño
General Surgery, Laproscopic Surgery
Address: Avenida Morones Prieto #3000
Poniente, Office #8
Borough: Colonia Los Doctores
Work: (81) 8143-0330, 8143-0440
Fax: (81) 8347-0500
Home: (81) 8378-5557
Mobiles: 044-81-8324-3355,
044-81-8063-7412
Email: fxtrevino@hotmail.com,
franciscot@hsj.com.mx
Pager: (81) 8151-1111, PIN# 56077

NEUROLOGISTS

Dr. David Del Pozo Reyes
Specializing In: Neurology
Autonomous University of Nuevo León,
1969 Centro Médico San José
Av. I. Morones Prieto # 3000 Poniente,
6th Floor, Room 610,
Col. Los Doctores, Monterrey
Office & Fax (81) 8347-1854
Home (81) 8303-0374
Cellular 044-811-509-5082
Email drdaviddelpozo@hotmail.com

OBSTETRICIAN

Dr. Carlos Félix
Obstetrics & Gynecology
Address: Calle "Dr. Cantú" #300, 5th floor

Borough: Colonia Los Doctores
Work/Fax: (81) 8333-3323
Home: (81) 8336-5404
Mobile: 044-81-8362-7036
Pager: (81) 8151-1111, PIN# 56598
Email: carfelar@infosel.net.mx

ONCOLOGISTS

Dr. Raymundo Diaz Mendoza
Hidalgo 2425
Col. Obispado, Monterrey
Tel: (81) 8347-5841 / 8318-6926
Dr. César González de León
Cerro de la Silla 815
Col. Obispado
Tel: (81) 8347-4821 / 24

OPHTHALMOLOGISTS

Dr. Enrique Barragán
Edificio Lorem, Planta Baja, Office 9
Hidalgo Pte. 2040 between Cerro de
Picachos and Emilio Zola
Col. Obispado, Monterrey
Tel: (81) 8348-6766 / 8004-0586

Dr. Rodrigo Garza Salinas
Washington Ote. 416-A
between Escobedo and Emilio Carranza
Col. Centro, Monterrey
Tel: (81) 8343-0196 / 8040-2425

Dr. Jesús Santiago Vidaurri Leal
Specializing In: Ophthalmology, Retina
Sub-Specialty
Autonomous University of Nuevo León,
1977 Centro Médico San José
Av. I. Morones Prieto # 3000 Poniente,
Room 901, Col. Los Doctores
Office Hours: 8-7:30
Office (81) 8333-5030 / 31 / 32
(81) 8151-3600 & 8333-5541
Fax (81) 8333-4601
Home (81) 8363-0844

Dr. Rogelio Villarreal Villareal
Centro de Oftalmologia Monterrey
Degollado 306 Sur
Colonia Maria Luisa
Tel: (81) 8675-6891 / 92 / 8346-2007
Fax: (81) 8675-6893
Website:
www.cirugialaserdeojos.blogspot.com

ORTHOPEDISTS

Dr. Humberto Criollos Flores
Specializing In: Orthopedics
University of San Luis Potosí, 1952
Centro Médico San José
Av. Morones Prieto # 3000,
Planta Baja, Room 10,
Col. Los Doctores, Monterrey
Office Hours: 10-12 4-6
Office (81) 8347-1024
Fax (81) 8348-0239
Home (81) 8303-1946

Dr. José Fernando De la Garza
Specializing In: Orthopedics,
Traumatologist
Autonomous University of Nuevo León,
1977 Centro Medico San José
Av. I. Morones Prieto # 3000, 7th Floor,
Col. Los Doctores, Monterrey
Office (81) 8333-2033, 8333-2333
Fax (81) 8333-3396
Mobile: 044-81-8185-3322
Pager: (81) 8151-1111, PIN# 18077
Email: jfdelag@hsj.com.mx

Dr. Raymundo Gonzalez
José Benitez 2704
Col. Obispado
Tel: (81) 8333-1466
E-mail: rggqnl1@yahoo.com

Dr. Alberto Padilla
Centro Médico Muguerza, 3rd floor,
of. 301 Ave. Hidalgo 2527
Col. Obispado, Monterrey, N.L.
Tel: (81) 8348-1607

PEDIATRICIANS

Dr. Pedro Cantú Gámez
Centro Médico San José
Av. Morones Prieto # 3000, Room 502,
Col. Los Doctores, Monterrey
Hours: M-F 9:30am–1pm Sat. 10:30am–1pm
Office (81) 8347-0036, 8348-2975
Home (81) 8338-1783

Dr. Alfonso E. Garza Rodríguez
Specializing In: Pediatrics
Autonomous University of Nuevo León,
1966 Centro Médico Hospital San José
Av. I. Morones Prieto # 3000, Room 301,
Col. Los Doctores, Monterrey
Office (81) 8348-2548, 8348-2549
(81) 8348-3081
Fax (81) 8347-4984
Home (81) 8333-3852
Email pedriatrasasociados@prodigy.net.mx

Dr. Francisco G. Lozano
Pediatrics
Address: Avenida Morones Prieto
#3000 Poniente
Borough: Colonia Los Doctores
Work: (81) 8348-2548, 8348-2549
Fax: (81) 8347-4984
Pager: (81) 8380-4500, PIN# 18382
Email: pediatras_asociados@prodigy.net.mx

Dr. Enrique Mendoza
Ave. La Clinica 2520, 3rd floor, Of. 310
Col. Sertoma, Monterrey,
Tel: (81) 8348-5701

Pediatras Asociados:
Dr. Francisco Lozano Lee,
Dr. Mario Dueñas Velasco,
Dr. José A. Lozano Villarreal,
Dr. Alfonso Garza Rodriguez,
Dr. Oscar Valencia
Centro Médico del Hospital San José
Av. Morones Prieto # 3000, 3rd Floor,
Room 301,
Col. Los Doctores,
Office (81) 8348-2548/49, 8348-3081

(81) 8348-2081
Emergencies Cellular 044-818-254-2517
Email pediatrasasociados@prodigy.net.mx

PLASTIC SURGEONS

Dr. Víctor Manuel Díaz Manjarrez
Autonomous University of Nuevo León,
1970 Centro Médico San José
Av. I. Morones Prieto # 3000 Poniente,
Rooms 208-2010,
Col. Los Doctores, Monterrey
Office (81) 8333-9292
Fax (81) 8346-0489
Cellular (81)8031-9210
Email vdiazmanjarrez@yahoo.com.mx

Dr. David Kirsch Kleiman
Autonomous University of Nuevo León,
1972 Edificio Delta Av. La Clínica # 2520,
Room 201,
Col. Sertoma, Monterrey
Office (81) 8346-5623, 8346-6317
Fax (81) 8347-2360
U.S. Based Phone 305-359-5377
Email drdavidk@intercable.net

Dr. Arnulfo Sepúlveda Nieto
University Of Monterrey, 1978
Centro Médico Metropolitano
Av. Del Hospital 110, Room 303,
Col. Sertoma, Monterrey
Office (81) 8348-9495
Cellular 044-818-253-4516
Home (81) 8336-4057
Email artesmedicas@live.com.mx

PHYSICAL THERAPISTS

Dr. Hernán C. Flores Carlos
University of Monterrey, 1976
Centro Médico San José
Av. I. Morones Prieto # 3000 Poniente,
7th Floor, Room 703,
Col. Los Doctores, Monterrey
Office (81) 8348-5584, 8348-1690

Hospital (81) 8347-1010 ext 2252
Email drhernan@hsj.com.mx

PSYCHIATRISTS / PSYCHOLOGISTS

Dr. Jesús Garza Perez
Autonomous University of Nuevo León, 1963
Centro Medico Inglés
Sertoma # 203 Sur, Room 402,
Col. Sertoma, Monterrey, Nuevo León,
Office Hours: 9-13 & 4-8
Office & Fax (81) 8333-1409
Cellular 044-811-545-2191
Email jgarzap@yahoo.com.mx

SPORTS MEDICINE

Dr. José Fernando De la Garza
Specializing In: Orthopedics,
Traumatologist
Autonomous University of Nuevo León,
1977 Centro Medico San José
Av. I. Morones Prieto # 3000, 7th Floor,
Col. Los Doctores, Monterrey
Office (81) 8333-2033, 8333-2333
Fax (81) 8333-3396
Mobile: 044-81-8185-3322
Pager: (81) 8151-1111, PIN# 18077
Email: jfdelag@hsj.com.mx

TRAUMATOLOGISTS

Dr. José Fernando De la Garza
Specializing In: Orthopedics,
Traumatologist
Autonomous University of Nuevo León,
1977 Centro Medico San José
Av. I. Morones Prieto # 3000, 7th Floor,
Col. Los Doctores, Monterrey
Office (81) 8333-2033, 8333-2333
Fax (81) 8333-3396
Mobile: 044-81-8185-3322
Pager: (81) 8151-1111, PIN# 18077
Email: jfdelag@hsj.com.mx

UROLOGISTS

Dr. Luis Fernando Guzmán De La Garza
Specializing In: Urology, Pediatric Urology
Autonomous University of Nuevo León
Centro Médico San José
Av. I. Morones Prieto # 3000 Poniente,
Consultorio 106,
Col. Los Doctores Monterrey
Office Hours: 4-8
Office & Fax (81) 8348-0659 & 8143-0109
Radio (81) 4774-1111 clave 542212
Home (81) 8363-1264

Dr. Angel Martínez Villarreal
Specializing In: Urology
Autonomous University of Nuevo León, 1968
Centro Médico San José
Av. I. Morones Prieto # 3000 Poniente,
1st Floor, Room 101,
Col. Los Doctores, Monterrey
Office (81) 8348-1291, 8348-2711
Radio (81) 8333-3152
Home (81) 8356-2529
Email consulmedic1@hotmail.com

HOSPITALS

Centro de Diagnóstico de Monterrey, S.C
Dr. Cantú # 300,
Col. Los Doctores, Monterrey
Telephone (81) 8348-6260, 8346-9000 to 09
Fax (81) 8347-5123

Centro de Especialidades Medicas
José Benitez 2704
Col. Obispado, Monterrey
Tel: (81) 8333-1466 / 8220-4444

Centro Médico Obispado
Hidalgo # 2530 Poniente,
Col. Obispado, Monterrey
Telephone (81) 8333-5049, 8346-7845,
(81) 8346-7858 & 8346-8448

Centro Médico Quirúrgico Irlandés
Sertoma # 105,
Col. Sertoma, Monterrey
Telephone (81) 8333-6632, 8333-6033,
8333-1213 & 8333-6631

Centro Profesional Delta
Ave. La Clínica # 2520,
Col. Los Doctores, Monterrey
Telephone (81) 8348-2935

Clínica Monterrey
Padre Mier 321 Poniente & Pino Suárez
Col. Centro, Monterrey
Telephone (81) 8343-2050 to 59

Hospital Christus Muguerza Conchita
15 de Mayo # 1822 Poniente,
Col. María Luisa, Monterrey, Nuevo León, Telephone (81) 8122-8122

Hospital Christus Muguerza Monterrey
Ave. Hidalgo 2525 Pte.
Col. Obispado, Monterrey
Tel: (81) 8399-3400
Emergencies: (81) 8399-3449 / 3453
Toll free: 01-800-557-2583
Website: www.christusmuguerza.com.mx

Hospital Christus Muguerza Sur
Carretera Nacional 6501
Col. La Estanzuela, Monterrey
Tel: (81) 8155-5000
Website: www.christusmuguerza.com.mx

Doctors Hospital
Ecuador # 2331,
Col. Balcones de Galerías, Monterrey
Telephone (81) 5515-5000
Hospital San José Tec de Monterrey
Ave. Ignacio Morones Prieto 3000
Col. Los Doctores, Monterrey,
Tel: (81) 8347-1010, 8115-1515
Emergencies: (81) 8347-1011, 8348-1010
Website: www.hsj.com.mx

Hospital San Lucas de Monterrey
Ave. La Clínica # 2565,
Col. Sertoma, Monterrey
Telephone (81) 8348-88-67, 8348-87-73
(81) 1052-3428, 1052-3439

Hospital San Vicente
Av. Ruperto Martinez Poniente # 1200,
Col. Centro, Monterrey
Telephone (81) 8345-7717, 8345-7777

Hospital Y Clinica OCA
Ave. Pino Suárez 645
Col. Centro, Monterrey
Tel: (81) 8262-0000
Emergencies: (81) 8289-0270
Website: www.ocahospital.com.mx

Hospital Universitario
Ave. Francisco I. Madero, corner
with Gonzalitos
Col. Mitras Sur, Monterrey
Tel: (81) 8389-1111
Emergencies: (81) 8388-1161 / 8389-1160
Website: www.medicina.uanl.mx

Hospital y Sanatorio Montemorelos
La Carlota (a.k.a. Centro Médico
Montemorelos)
Camino Al Vapor # 209,
Col. Centro (four blocks from Carretera
Nacional) Montemorelos,
Telephone (826) 263-3188, 263-3404, 263-3328, (826) 263-3060, 63-3425 & 263-3430

MORELIA

GYNECOLOGISTS

Dr. Manuel Eduardo Ayala Tames
General Pedro Ampudia 55
Col. Chapultepec
Morelia, Michoacán
Tel: (443) 204-4343
Cell: (443) 164-6851

Dr. Jorge Zepeda-Ortéga
Obstetrics & Gynecology
Address: Calle Virrey de Mendóza
#1998, Office 004
Borough: Colonia Félix Ireta
Work/Fax: (443) 340-5003
Mobile: 044-443-202-1086
Email: zepedamd@aol.com

INTERNISTS

Dr. Francisco Eduardo Quintana
Internal Medicine, Nephrology
Address: Calle Virrey de Mendóza
#1998, Office 614
Borough: Colonia Félix Ireta
Work/Fax: (443) 324-0581, 299-2847
Mobile: 044-443-318-4929
Email: qupdiaz@hotmail.com

NEPHROLOGISTS

Dr. Francisco Eduardo Quintana
Internal Medicine, Nephrology
Address: Calle Virrey de Mendóza
#1998, Office 614
Borough: Colonia Félix Ireta
Work/Fax: (443) 324-0581, 299-2847
Mobile: 044-443-318-4929
Email: qupdiaz@hotmail.com

OBSTETRICIANS

Dr. Manuel Eduardo Ayala Tames
General Pedro Ampudia 55
Col. Chapultepec, Morelia, Michoacán
Tel: (443) 204-4343
Cell: (443) 164-6851

Dr. Jorge Zepeda-Ortéga
Obstetrics & Gynecology
Address: Calle Virrey de Mendóza
#1998, Office 004
Borough: Colonia Félix Ireta
Work/Fax: (443) 340-5003
Mobile: 044-443-202-1086
Email: zepedamd@aol.com

PEDIATRICIANS

Dr. Jorge A. Vázquez
Pediatrics, Pediatrics Infectious Disease
Address: Calle Virrey de Mendóza
#1998, Office 401
Borough: Colonia Félix Ireta
Work: (443) 324-5436
Mobile: 044-443-310-1411
Nextel: 1654516
Home: (443) 324-7065
Email: fix55@msn.com

UROLOGISTS

Dr. Roberto Fonseca
Address: Calle Virrey de Mendóza
#1998, Office 500
Borough: Colonia Félix Ireta
Work: (443) 299-3080
Mobile: 044-443-155-1537
Email: rfonsecadoc@yahoo.com.mx

HOSPITALS

Clínica Médica de Morelia
Av. Lázaro Cárdenas 2020
Col. Chapultepec, Morelia, Michoacán
Tel: (443) 314-3807

Cruz Roja
Calzada Ventura Puente 27
Col. Centro, Morelia, Michoacán
Tel: (443) 314-5025/5245

Hospital Acueducto
Ave. Acueducto 581
Col. Vasco de Quiroga
Morelia, Michoacán
Tel: (443) 324-8402 / 03 / 04
E-mail: info@hospitalacueducto.com
Website: www.hospitalacueducto1.com

Hospital Clínica Universidad
Av. Universidad 745
Morelia, Michoacán
Tel: (443) 326-2913 / 5675

Hospital General "Dr. Miguel Silva"
Isidro Huarte
corner with Samuel Ramos
Col. Centro, Morelia, Michoacán
Tel: (443) 312-0102/ 317-2216

Hospital Nueva España
Samuel Ramos 557
Col. Centro, Morelia, Michoacán
Tel: (443) 312-4548 / 9553

Hospital Star Médica
Virrey de Mendoza 2000
Col. Feliz Ireta, Morelia, Michoacán
Tel: (443) 322-7700
Emergencies: (443) 322-7700 ext. 1034
Website: www.starmedica.com.mx

Sanatorio Cuautla
Cuautla 788
Col. Molino de Parras, Morelia, Michoacán
Tel: (443) 312-1067 / 4278 / 317-4496

Sanatorio La Luz
General Bravo 50
Col. Chapultepec Norte, Morelia, Michoacán
Tel: (443) 315-2966 / 2967
Fax: (443) 315-2968
Website: www.sanatoriolaluz.com

NAUCALPAN

HOSPITAL

Hospital Angeles de Interlomas
Av. Vialidad de la Barranca
(no street number)
Col. Valle de las Palmas, Huixquilucan
Estado. de Mexico
5246-50-00 5246-50-93 5246-50-92

VETERINARIANS

Dr. Rafael Maya
Avenida de las Fuentes 174, local 51
Tecamachalco, Naucalpan, Estado de México
Tel: (55) 5589-2958
Cell: (55) 9166-0265
Hours: Monday-Friday, 10-14 and 16-19
Saturday, 10-14

NAVAOJOA

ALLERGISTS

Dr. Armando Carvajal Chavez
Calle Otero 205 Sur Immunology
Colonia Reforma,Navojoa, Sonora
Phone: (642) 422-0751

CARDIOLOGISTS

Dr. Jairo Enriquez
Clinica de Especialidades
No Reeleccion y Bravo #616 sur, Dep. 2
Navojoa, Sonora
Phone/Fax: (642) 422-7955
E-Mail: jairoenriquez@hotmail.com

EAR, NOSE & THROAT

Dr. Miguel Enrique Felix Sanz
Obregon y Otero No. 216 Dept. C
Navojoa, Sonora,
Phone: (642) 422-4828,
Fax: (642) 421-3072
E-Mail: miguel_e_felix@hotmail.com

GASTROENTEROLOGIST

Dr. Joaquin Ricardo Flores Perez
Ave. Quintana Roo #300
Entre Toledo y Rincón
Navojoa, Sonora
Phone/Fax: (642) 422-1310, (642) 421-4979
E-Mail: drjrfp@hotmail.com

INTERNISTS

Dr. Danilo Manuel Gonzalez Roman
Central Biomédica
Quintana Roo #104 Oriente
Colonia Centro, Navojoa, Sonora,
Phone: (642) 422-5755, 422-7402,
422-1026
Email: drdanilogonzalez@hotmail.com

OPHTALMOLOGISTS

Dr. Julio Manuel Martinez Almada
Av. Hidalgo #106 Poniente
Colonia Reforma, Navojoa, Sonora
Phone: (642) 422-4300, 422-0667
Email: jmtzalmada@hotmail.com

Dr. Javier Rojas Cañez
Obregon y Rincon #402
Navojoa, Sonora,
Phone/Fax: (642) 422-7262
E-Mail: chilorojas@hotmail.com

ORTHOPEDICIANS

Dr. Gustavo Acosta Gaxiola
Traumatology
Clinica San Jose
Ave. Sosa Chavez #302
Navojoa, Sonora,
Phone: (642) 422-1026
E-Mail: acostaggustavo@hotmail.com

Dr. Raul Garcia Garcia
Traumatology & Orthopedics
No Reeleccion #515 Sur
Navojoa, Sonora,
Phone/Fax: (642) 422-8282,
(642) 422-7413
Home: (642) 422-6606
Email: drraulgarciagarcia@hotmail.com

HOSPITALS

Clinica Hospital San Jose de Navojoa
Ave. Sosa Chávez #302 poniente
Navojoa, Sonora,
Phone: (642) 422-7401, (642) 422-1026

Sanatorío Lourdes
Calle No Reeleccion 504 Sur
on the corner of Quintana Roo
Navojoa, Sonora,
Phone: (642) 422-0200, (642) 422-1407
Phone: (642) 422-9043, (642) 422-9044
Email: atencion@sanatoriolourdes.org

NUEVO LAREDO

CARDIOLOGISTS

Dr. Miguel Jaime Garcia-Rojas Armengol,
Address: 15 de Septiembre #34
Phone: 715-0515 & 714-6808

DERMATOLOGISTS

Dra. Alejandra Daw Garza,
Address: Tax.co #3639-A
Phone: 714-2150

Dr. Luz Marcela Vidaurri Souza,
Address: Carnpeche #2333, Suite 2
Phone: 715-6826

EAR, NOSE & THROAT

Dr. Liliana Arjona Barocio,
Specialty: Otorhinolaryngologist
Address: Juarez #2713
Phone: 715-2964

Dr. Julio Cesar De La Rosa Trevino,
Specialty: Otorhinolaryngologist
Address: Baja California #3405
Phone: 715-5664

Dr. Misael Rodriguez Garza, Misael,
Dr. Misael Rodriguez Vazquez, Misael,
Specialties: Otorhinolaryngology & Nasal
Sinuses Endoscopic Surgery Specialist.
Address: Ocampo #3014
Phone: 714-9202 & 714-1233

FAMILY MEDICINE

Dr. Carlos Barreto Lepe, Carlos,
Address: Nuevo Leon #2212
Specialty: Family Medicine
Phone: 715-3268

Dr. Agustin Tomas Saldana Asunsolo,
Address: Gutierrez #260 1
Specialty: Family Medicine
Phone: 712-2580

GENERAL MEDICINE

Dr. Luis Evaristo Martinez Salgado,
Address: Obregon #2402
Phone: 715-0016

Dr. Homero Vela Salinas
Address: Gonzalez #5504
Phone: 712-8900

GASTROENTEROLOGISTS

Dr. Jesus Arturo Armenta Jasso,
Address: Baja California #3401
Phone: 715-9305

Dr. Cesar Omar Ortega Vela,
Specialties: Internal Medicine &
Gastroenterologist
Address: Aquiles Serdan #3135
Phone:714-1740

GYNECOLOGISTS

Dra. Ana Laura Cardenas Thomae,
Address: Orizaba #3752
Phone: 719-2200

Dr. Guadalupe Rebeca, Diaz Vazquez,
Address: Baja California #2526
Phone: 715-7000

Dr. Rodolfo Garcia Morales,
Address: Obregon #2402
Phone: 715-2121

Dr. Amparo Lepe Galindo,
Address: Nuevo Leon #2212
Phone: 715-3268

Dr. Juan Manuel Ramirez Garcia,
Address: Reynosa #3002
Phone: 714-0510

HEMATOLOGISTS

Dr. Cristina, Tovar Martinez,
Address: Baja California #340 1
Phone: 711-2020

INTERNISTS

Dr. Mario Alberto Arreola Herrera,
Specialties: Internal Medicine & Infections
Address: Guerrero #3005
Phone: 711-2900

Dr. Dagoberto Martinez Benavides,
Address: Chihuahua #2507
Phone: 715-7487

Dr. Cesar Omar Ortega Vela,
Specialties: Internal Medicine &
Gastroenterologist
Address: Aquiles Serdan #3135
Phone:714-1740

ONCOLOGISTS

Dr. Hugo Rene Ortega Vela,
Specialties: General Surgeon & Oncologist
Address: Aquiles Serdan #3135
Phone: 714-1740

OPHTALMOLOGISTS

Dr. Francisco Javier Fragoso Garcia,
Address: Morelos #21 06
Phone: 714-2761 & 711-7882

Garcia Gonzalez, Misael, Dr.
Address: Ocampo #3428
Phone: 714-9080 & 714-0667

Dr. Gerardo Gascon Iturralde,
Dr. Gerardo Gascon Guzman,
Specialties: Ophthalmologist & Retina
Specialist.
Address: Morelos #2813
Phone: 714-9040

Vazquez Gonzalez, Modesto, Dr.
Address: Chihuahua #2958
Phone: 715-4600

ORTHOPEDIST / TRAUMATOLOGISTS

Dr. Gerardo Cesar Garcia Aguilar,
Address: Ocampo #31 09
Phone: 714-4486

Dr. Mario Alberto Perez Coss,
Address: Gonzalez #5504
Phone: 712-8900
Emergency: 011-521-867-156-9667

Dr. Francisco Javier Ramirez Pompa,
Address: Dr. Mier #1812
Phone: 712-1478

Dr. Carlos Alberto Sosa Santillan,
Address: Morelos #2846
Phone: 710-0934

Dr. Leonel Vazquez Salinas,
Address: Dr. Mier #3636
Phone: 712-1670 & 712-4272

PEDIATRICIANS

Dra. Maria del Rosario Acosta Medina,
Address: 15 de Septiembre #34
Phone: 715-0515 & 714-6808

Dr. Maximo Eduardo Contreras Santiago,
Address: Baja California #2526
Phone: 715-7000

Dr. Mario Luis Pineda Maldonado,
Dr. Mario Luis, Pineda Pinto,
Specialties: Allergist & Pediatrician
Address: Maclovio Herrera # 1940
Phone: 712-3420

Dr. Juan Carlos Takasita,
Address: Nuevo Leon #2212
Phone: 715-5191 & 715-3268

Dr. Juana Alicia Vazquez Cruz,
Address: Obregon #3161
Phone: 714-0174

PSYCHIATRISTS

Dr. Isidro Demencio Caballero Jimenez,
Address: Oceano Pacifico #536
Specialty: Psychiatrist
Phone: 715-5797

RADIOLOGISTS

Dr. Armando Echavarria,
Address: Aquiles Serdan #2020
Phone: 714-7453 &715-0592

Dr. Octaviano Martinez,
Address: Aquiles Serdan #2020
Phone: 714-7453 & 715-0592

RHEUMATOLOGISTS

Dr.Hermann E Muñoz Monsivais,
Address: Juarez #3004
Phone: 714-7698 & 714-9999

SURGEON

Dr. Jesus Gonzalez Cepeda,
Specialty: General Surgeon
Address: Baja California #3401
Phone: 711-2020

Dr. Abelardo Osuna Madrigal,
A Specialties: General Laparoscopic
Surgery & Obesity.
Address: Baja California #2526
Phone: 715-7581

UROLOGISTS

Crespo Nava, Oscar Gerardo, Dr.
Address: Maclovio Herrera #1940
Specialty: Urologist
Phone: 713-0505

HOSPITALS

Hospital San Jose
Guerrero 3003
714-9506 & 714-9076

Hospital de la Cruz Roja
Mexicana Comonfort e Independencia
712-0989 &712-0949

NOGALES

GENERAL MEDICINE

Dr. Jose Luis Castro Jr.
Dr. Hector Silva Platt
Central Medica de Especialidades Av.
Obregon No. 279
Av. Obregon No. 668-5 Col. Centro
Phone: (6) 312-51-21
Phone: (6) 312-4570

Dr. Jesus Enrique Bermudez Nunez
Dr. Heriberto Hernandez
Campillo 86 Despacho 204 Calle Diaz # 40
Phone: (6) 312-11-30 Phone &
Fax: (6) 312-5089

DENTISTS

Dr. Jesus Enrique Bermudez Nunez
Obregon # 436-2
Phone: (6) 312-4052

Dr. Ramon Ibarra Fontes
Obregon # 240, 2nd. Floor
Phone: (6) 312-2015

Dr. Miguel Angel Molina Medina
Dr. Adrain R. Molina Medina
P. Elias Calles 880 Local 9
Phone: (6) 313-5757
(Equipped with Dental Laboratory)

Dr. Fabian Rio Gonzalez
Pasaje Morelos No. 78 1st. Floor
Between Campillo & Ochoa
Phone: (6) 312-5357

HOSPITALS

Centro Medico de Sonora
Ana G. Guervara 71 (antes Campodonico)
Phone (631) 71, 3-0661 & 3-0916

Hospital del Socorro
Hermosillo # 425,
Phone (631) 4-60-60, 4-60-61

Hospital General (Seneson)
Calle Francisco Arriola #1277,
Phone: 313-0794; 313-3465

Hospital Sabta Teresa
Ingenieros # 407 Altos,
Phone (631) 2-45-60 & 2-05-06

OAXACA

CARDIOLOGISTS

Dr. Alejo Diaz Aragon
Juárez 504
Colonia Centro
Oaxaca, Oaxaca
Tel: (951) 514-9388
Cell: (951) 548-1896

DENTISTS

Dr. Angel Gomez
Bustamante 312-A
Colonia Centro
Oaxaca, Oaxaca
Tel: (951) 516-4959 / 4153
Fax: (951) 516-4153
E-mail: gomezagr@hotmail.com

Dr Rafael Enrique Madina Baños
Cielo 203
Colonia Lomas del Creston
Oaxaca, Oaxaca
Tel & Fax: (951) 513-9520
Emergency Cell: (951) 526-0603
E-mail: rafavol@hotmail.com

Dra. Martha Ortega
Escuela Naval Militar 402
Colonia Reforma
Oaxaca, Oaxaca
Tel: (951) 513-0413 / 518-4435

Dr. Daniel Tenorio Oda
Abasolo 213-3
Colonia Centro
Oaxaca, Oaxaca
Tel: (951) 516-2613

GENERAL MEDICINE

Dr. Marco Antonio
Calleja Sanchez
Belisario Dominguez 115
Colonia Reforma
Oaxaca, Oaxaca
Tel: (951) 515-3492

Dr. Javier Gutierrez Altamirano
Calzada Panteón Jardín 127, Casa 32
Fracc. Residencial Jazmines
San Andrés Huayapan
Oaxaca, Oaxaca
Tel: (951) 513-9917
Cell: (951) 118-6728
E-mail: drgut52@yahoo.com.mx

Dr. Enrique Robert Garcia
Priv. de Monte Albán 10
on Calzada Porfirio Diaz
Colonia Reforma
Oaxaca, Oaxaca
Tel: (951) 515-3459
Emergency Cell: (951) 183-0421

Dr. Horacio Tenorio Rodriguez
Abasolo 215
Colonia Centro
Oaxaca, Oaxaca
Tel: (951) 514-7545 / 516-2612 / 0027
Fax: (951) 516-0027
Email: gilo0719@hotmail.com

GERONTOLOGISTS

Dr. Horacio de Jesús Tenorio
General Medicine, Gerontology
Address: Calle Abasolo #215, Office 110
Borough: Colonia Centro
Work: (951) 514-7545
Fax: (951) 516-0027
Home: (951) 517-5779
Pager: 044-951-127-8856
Email: gilo0719@hotmail.com

GYNECOLOGISTS

Dra. Tzatzil Ayala Barahona
Clinica Santo Domingo
Alcala 808
Colonia Centro
Oaxaca, Oaxaca
Office hours: 10:30-12
Tel: (951) 513-2600

Dr. Victor L. Tenorio
Obstetrics & Gynecology
Address: Calle Abasolo #215
Borough: Colonia Centro
Work: (951) 514-2889
Fax: (951) 516-4468
Home: (951) 517-7842
Mobile: 044-951-128-1345
Email: victenvas@hotmail.com

INTERNISTS

Dr. Ramón Jiménez
Internal Medicine, Oncology
Address: Calle Emiliano Zapata #316,
Office 3
Borough: Colonia Reforma
Work: (951) 513-7440
Fax: (951) 515-7200
Home: (951) 520-0659
Mobile: 044-951-128-1234
Emergency Mobile: 044-951-147-5171
Email: drjimenezcaballero@hotmail.com

Dr. Sergio Molina
Internal Medicine
Address: Calle Xicotencatl #1019
Borough: Colonia Centro
Work: (951) 516-6249, 501-1308
Fax: (951) 501-1308
Mobile: 044-951-507-0012
Pager: 515-6800, PIN# 4450
Email: sergiomolina570106@hotmail.com

NEUROLOGISTS

Dr. Jorge Ayala Villareal
Clínica Santo Domingo
Alcalá 808
Colonia Centro
Oaxaca, Oaxaca
Tel: (951) 513-2600 / 513-0060
Home: (951) 515-2323
Office hours: 15-17, 20-22

OBSTETRICIANS

Dr. Victor L. Tenorio
Obstetrics & Gynecology
Address: Calle Abasolo #215
Borough: Colonia Centro
Work: (951) 514-2889
Fax: (951) 516-4468
Home: (951) 517-7842
Mobile: 044-951-128-1345
Email: victenvas@hotmail.com

ONCOLOGISTS

Dr. Ramón Jiménez
Internal Medicine, Oncology
Address: Calle Emiliano Zapata #316,
Office 3
Borough: Colonia Reforma
Work: (951) 513-7440
Fax: (951) 515-7200
Home: (951) 520-0659
Mobile: 044-951-128-1234
Emergency Mobile: 044-951-147-5171
Email: drjimenezcaballero@hotmail.com

PEDIATRICIANS

Dr. Rodolfo Garcia Caballero
Pediatrician and Allergist
Clínica Santo Domingo
Alcalá 808
Colonia Centro, Oaxaca, Oaxaca
Tel: (951) 513-2600

Dra. Rosa Garcia Muñoz
Pediatrician and Allergist
Clínica de Pediatría, Asma y Alergias SC
Calzada Madero 108
Colonia Centro
Oaxaca, Oaxaca
Tel: (951) 516-3750

Dr. Carlos Pacheco Skidmore
Humboldt 205, corner with Quintana Roo
Colonia Centro, Oaxaca, Oaxaca
Tel: (951) 516-3943
Cell: (951) 102-1414
Office hours: 11-14:30, 18-20

Dr. Hector Tenorio Rodriguez
Unidad Pediátrica Privada
Alamos 607
Colonia Reforma, Oaxaca, Oaxaca
Tel: (951) 513-3890 / 5355
E-mail: hecter84@hotmail.com

TRAUMATOLOGISTS

Dr. Hector Rodriguez Castro
Eucaliptos 401, corner with Amapolas
Colonia Reforma, Oaxaca, Oaxaca
Tel & Fax: (951) 515-4533

UROLOGISTS

Dr. Antonio Sanchez Vega
Hospital Molina
García Vigil 317
Colonia Centro, Oaxaca, Oaxaca
Tel: (951) 514-2050 / 516-3836

HOSPITALS - PRIVATE

Centro Medico de Traumatologia y Ortopedia
Clínica Hospital Florencia
Curtidurías 320
Barrio de Jalatlaco, Oaxaca, Oaxaca
Tel & Fax: (951) 513-6884 / 518-6926

Clínica Hospital Carmen
Address: Calle Abasolo #215 (between
Avenida Reforma and Avenida Juárez)
Borough: Zona Centro
Notable Landmarks: Regional Museum and St.
Domingo Church
Main Phone #: (951) 516-2612
Fax Phone #: (951) 516-0027

Hospital Reforma
Reforma 613
Colonia Centro
Notable Landmarks: Regional Museum
and Santo Domingo Church
Oaxaca, Oaxaca
Tel: (951) 516-0989
Tel. & Fax: (951) 514-6277

Médica 2002
Address: Calle Emiliano Zapata #316
Borough: Colonia Reforma
(northern part of town)
Notable Landmarks: University of Oaxaca Medi-
cal School
Main Phone #: (951) 515-7200
Fax Phone #: (951) 513-1169

Sanatorío del Carmen
Abasolo 215
Colonia Centro, Oaxaca, Oaxaca
Tel: (951) 516-2612 / 514-7545
Fax: (951) 516-0027

Sanatorío Molina
García Vigil 317
Colonia Centro, Oaxaca, Oaxaca
Tel: (951) 516-5468

PALENQUE

GENERAL MEDICINE

Dr. Alfonso Martínez
Address: Avenida Dr. Velasco Suárez #33
Work: (916) 345-0273
Home/Fax: (916) 345-1513

HOSPITAL

Cruz Roja
Between Maca and Caoba
Colonia Luis Donaldo Colosio
Palenque, Chiapas
Tel: (916) 345-4154

PATZCUARO

HOSPITALS

Centro de Salud
Lloreda Nueva (no street number)
Patzcuaro, Michoacán
Tel: (434) 342-0884

Hospital General "Dr. Gabriel García"
Romero (no street number)
Patzcuaro, Michoacán
Tel: (434) 342-0285

PLAYA DEL CARMEN

ALTERNATIVE MEDICINE

Dr. Luis David Suarez Rodriguez,
General Medicine, Acupuncture and Ozone
Treatments.
Phone: 803-2039,
Sanar.sc@gmail.com

ANESTHESIOLOGIST

Dra. Marisela Jimenez Contreras,
Hospiten,
Phone: 803-1002

Dr. Roberto Lazo,
Costamed,
Phone: 803-7777

Dr. Rigoberto Pelagio Pena,
Costamed,
cell 116-3106.

CARDIOLOGISTS

Dr. Gustavo Lopez Nava,
Phone: 803-8620,
Nextel cell: 998-185-4614

Dr. Vladmir Heriberto Ruiz Ronquillo,
Phone: 109-5613,
Cell: 114-5552 or 219-1740

Dr. Omar David Santoyo Pacheco,
Hospiten,
Phone: 803-1002

COLPOSCOPY

Dra. Linda Velasco
Obstetrics & Gynecology, Colposcopy
Address: Avenida Constituyentes
(between Calle 10 and Calle 15),
Mza. 62, Lote 5, Local 3
Borough: Colonia Centro
Work: (984) 803-3517
Mobile: 044-984-128-7883
Email: linda.velasco@hotmail.com

DENTISTS

Dr. Esteban Barragan
Bokanova Dental Center
Plaza Paraiso Caribe
Ave. 10 Sur, entre Calle 3 y 5 Sur
Col. Centro, Playa del Carmen, Q.Roo
Tel: (984) 803-1043
Cell: (777) 279-7583

Coral Dental Center,
Av. Juarez with Calle 25,
Centro, Playa del Carmen,
Phone: 803 – 1622,
Emergencies: 876-2839

Dra. Maria de la Luz Pali Herrera,
Calle 4 #230 Local 1 /
between 30 Av and 35 Av,
Centro, Playa del Carmen,
Phone: 873-2429,
Emergencies: 100-5992

Dr. Perla Rocha Torres,
Phone: 803-2429,
Emergencies: 106-1276

EAR, NOSE & THROAT

Dr. Giorge H. J. Humberto.
Hospiten,
Phone: 803-1002 or 01-800-101-2255

Dra. Magali Gonzalez Gutierez,
Costamed,
Phone: 803-7777

Dr. J. Federico Williamson
Address: Calle Balamcanche,
Mza. 30,Lote1
Borough: Playacar fase II
Work: (984) 803-1002
Fax: (984) 803-1606
Mobile: 01-998-845-1052
Email: fwilliamson@hospiten.com

GENERAL MEDICINE

Dr. Roberto Amora.
Costamed,
Phone: 803-7777

Dr. Rodrigo Blasco Figueroa,
Hospiten,
Phone: 803-1002

Dra. Maria del Carmen Fernandez Perez,
Hospiten Riviera Maya
Phone: 803-1002

Dr. Juan Antonio Fonseca Ordonoz,
Hospiten,
Phone: 803-1002

Dra Pavlova Gaxiola,
Costamed,
Phone: 803-7777

César I. Ramírez
General Medicine
Address: Avenida 15 Norte #16
(between Calle 38 and 40)
Borough: Fraccionamiento Zacil-Ha
Work/Fax: (984) 803-6194, 859-4693
Mobile: 044-984-876-2175

Dr. Misael Rivas Lopez,
Hospiten,
Phone: 803-7777

Dr. José E. Rovirosa
General Medicine, Hyperbaric Medicine,
Subaquatic andDiving Medicine
Address: Avenida 10, #329,
at the corner of Calle 28 North
Work: (984) 873-1365, 803-1216
Fax: (984) 873-1755
Mobile: 044-984-804-7839
Email: rovirosamd@hotmail.com

Dr. Citlaly Rubalcaba,
Costamed,
Phone: 803-7777

GYNECOLOGISTS

Dr. Mauricio Isaac Canul Rojas,
Hospiten,
Phone: 803-1002,
Cell: 116-4747

Dr. Muriel Pliego,
Hospiten,
Phone: 803- 1002,
Cell: 134-2001

Dra. Linda Velasco
Obstetrics & Gynecology, Colposcopy
Address: Avenida Constituyentes
(between Calle 10 and Calle 15),
Mza. 62, Lote 5, Local 3
Borough: Colonia Centro
Work: (984) 803-3517
Mobile: 044-984-128-7883
Email: linda.velasco@hotmail.com

HYPERBARIC MEDICINE

Dr. José E. Rovirosa
General Medicine, Hyperbaric Medicine,
Subaquatic and Diving Medicine
Address: Avenida 10, #329,
at the corner of Calle 28 North
Work: (984) 873-1365, 803-1216
Fax: (984) 873-1755
Mobile: 044-984-804-7839
Email: rovirosamd@hotmail.com

INTERNISTS

Dr. Eduardo Chavez Marquez,
Costamed,
Phone: 803-7777

Dr. Oscar Hernandez Gea,
Hospiten,
Phone: 803 – 1002

Dr. Rafael Maciel Morfin,
Clinica del Carmen,
Costamed, Playamed, Sacbe Clinic,
Cell: 168-6785
Email: Rafael@starnuero.com

OBSTETRICIANS

Dra. Linda Velasco
Obstetrics & Gynecology, Colposcopy
Address: Avenida Constituyentes
(between Calle 10 and Calle 15),
Mza. 62, Lote 5, Local 3
Borough: Colonia Centro
Work: (984) 803-3517
Mobile: 044-984-128-7883
Email: linda.velasco@hotmail.com

ORTHOPEDISTS

Dr. Luis Demetrio Amaro Lopez,
Playamed,
Phone: 879-3145 or 3147,
Cell: 801-7818
Email: dr_idamaro@hotmail.com

Dr. Fernando Corona Gomez,
Costamed, Phone: 803-7777,
Nextel cell: 155-2478
coronatrauma@gmail.com

Dr. Carlos Cuervo Cruz,
Hospiten,
Phone: (984) 803-1002,
Juancarlos.cuervo@hospiten.com

Dr. Ricardo Galvan Martinez,
Cell: 801-5638,
Email: drgalvan@cartilago,
www.cartilago.net

PEDIATRICIANS

Dr. Daniel Bueno Saavedra,
Hospiten,
Phone: 803-1002

Dra. Beatriz Gutierrez Medina /
Dr. Sergio Meniovich,
UNID Building, Carretera Fed. with Calle 28
Ejido, Playa del Carmen, QRoo,
Phone: 803-8329,
Cell: 876-2683 / 125-7053

Dr. Carlos Rosado,
Costamed,
Phone: 803-7777

PSYCHIATRISTS

Psic. Leslie David (Therapist),
Cell: 113-4113
www.psicoterapiasobreruedas.com

Dr. Jorge Polanco Benois
30 Av. Nte Lote 4 Apt. 4 /
between Calle 30 and Calle 32
Playa del Carmen, QROO
Phone: 873-3347,
Cell: 876-2337
Jpolancob@hotmail.com

RADIOLOGISTS

Best Medical Diagnostic Center,
Carr. Fed. with Av Juarez
(Next to Banorte),
Phone: 803-9363 or 9364

Dr. Carlos Adolfo Velasco Ospina,
Hospiten,
Phone: 803-1002

DIVING MEDICINE

Dr. José E. Rovirosa
General Medicine, Hyperbaric Medicine,
Subaquatic and Diving Medicine
Address: Avenida 10, #329,
at the corner of Calle 28 North
Work: (984) 873-1365, 803-1216
Fax: (984) 873-1755
Mobile: 044-984-804-7839
Email: rovirosamd@hotmail.com

UROLOGISTS

Dr. Ernesto Alfonso Diaz Garcia,
Hospiten,
Phone: 803-1002

HOSPITALS

Buceo Médico Mexicano
Hyperbaric Chamber Facility
Address: Avenida 10 #329
(on the corner of Calle 28)
Colonia Centro
Playa del Carmen,
Quintana Roo
Main Phone #: (984) 873-1365
Fax Phone #: (984) 873-1755

Clinica Medica del Carmen
Ave. 25 between Calle 2 Norte and
Avenida Benito Juárez
(next to Bancomer bank)
Colonia Centro
Playa del Carmen, Quintana Roo
Tel: (984) 873-0885 / 803-1442
Fax: (984) 873-0885
http://www.medicadelcarmen.com/

Clinica Sacbe
Calle 34 bis. / 30 Av y 35 Av,
Playa del Carmen,
QRoo, ,
Phone: 803-0055, 873-1576
clinicasacbe@yahoo.com.mx

Emergencies 24 hours,
Services:Ultrasounds, Laparoscopic
Surgery, Birthing Center, General Surgery,
X-Rays. Clinical Laboratories
Martinez & Arcila, Av Juarez
between Av 45 and Carr. Fed.,
Centro, Playa del Carmen, QRoo,
Phone: 873-0633, 803-0140,
Cell: 115-4446
Email: qfbdoris@prodigy.net.mx

Grupo Medico Costamed
Edificio Progreso, Planta Baja
(before Centro Maya)
Carretera Federal, Mza. 285, Lt. 7
between 27 and 23
Colonia Ejido Sur
Playa del Carmen, Quintana Roo
Tel: (984) 803-7777/ 9825
http://costamed.com.mx/welcome/our-facilities/
playa-del-carmen-facility/

Hospital General
Ave. Constituyentes and Calle 135
Colonia Ejidal
Playa del Carmen, Quintana Roo
Tel: (984) 206-1690 to 92

Hospital Hospiten – Riviera Maya
Address: Calle Balamcanche,
Mza. 30, Lote1
Borough: Playacar fase II
Phone: (984) 803-1002
Fax: (984) 803-1606

Hospital Playa Med
Carretera Federal
Calle 28 Norte, Mza. 4, Lote 4
(next to the appliance store Telebodega)
Colonia Ejidal
Playa del Carmen, Quintana Roo
Tel: (984) 879-3155 / 3143 / 3145

Hospital San Carlos
Carretera Federal Mza. 155, Lote 3
Col. Ejido Sur, Playa del Carmen, Q. Roo
Tel: (984) 859-3313
E-mail: hospitalsancarlos@prodigy.net.mx

Hospiten Riviera Maya
Calle Balamcanche Mza. 30, Lote 1
(Second entrance to Condominio Playacar II)
Col. Centro, Playa del Carmen, Q. Roo
Tel: (984) 803-1002
Fax: (984) 803-1016
E-mail: rivieramaya@hospiten.com
http://www.hospiten.com/en/centro/hospiten-
riviera-maya

PIEDRAS NEGRAS

ALLERGISTS

Dr. Rafael Acosta Ortiz,
Address: Morelos #205 11
Phone: 782-2524

GYNECOLOGISTS

Dra. Artemisa Cadena,
Address: 16 de Septiembre #804
Phone: 782-3050

Dr. Carlos Daniel Martinez Garcia,
Address: 16 de Septiembre #804
Phone:782-5620

INTERNISTS

Dr. Jorge Luis Munoz Viguera,
Address: Teran #401 Oriente, Suite 23
Specialty: Internal Medicine
Phone: 782-4888

ORTHOPEDISTS

Gonzalez Olivares, Eduardo, Dr.
Address: Teran #401 C15
Specialty: Orthopedist
Phone: 782-1626

PEDIATRICIANS

Roiz Reyes, Arturo, Dr.
Address: Teran #113 Poniente
Specialty: Pediatrician
Phone: 782-4180

RHEUMATOLOGIST

Munoz De Hoyos, Jorge Luis, Dr.
Address: Teran #401 Oriente, Suite A
Specialties: Rheumatologist, Clinical
Immunology & Internal Medicine
Phone: 782-2333

SURGEON

Gonzalez Guajardo, Gabriel, Dr.
Address: Teran #113 Poniente
Specialty: General Laparoscopic Surgery
Phone: 782-8135
U.S. Phone: 830-776-3287

TRAUMATOLOGISTS

Castro Rodriguez, Omar, Dr.
Address: Teran #113 Poniente
Specialty: Traumatologist
Phone: 782-4180

Mondragon Ritchie, Manuel, Dr.
Address: Teran #111
Specialty: Traumatologist
Phone: 782-4553

Munguia Robles, Jorge Eduardo, Dr.
Address: Teran #113 Poniente
Specialty: Traumatologist
Phone: 782-4180

UROLOGISTS

Campos Amescua, Bertin, Dr.
Address: Teran #113 Poniente
Specialty: Urologist
Phone: 782-4180

HOSPITALS

Clinica de Especialistas
E. Carranza 1017
Piedras Negras, Coahuila
Tel: (878) 782-1297 / 5464

Clinica Maternidad Lupita
Colon 212 Oriente
Colonia Centro
Piedras Negras, Coahuila
Tel: (878) 782-4666

Clinica San Jose
Teran 115 Poniente
Colonia Centro
Piedras Negras, Coahuila
Tel: (878) 782-5551

Hospital Civil Municipal
Emilio Carranza 1202
Colonia Piedras Negras
Piedras Negras, Coahuila
Tel: (878) 782-2973

PROGRESO

GENERAL MEDICINE

Dr. Sergio Bates
General Medicine
Address: Calle 33 #320
(at the corner of Calle 82)
Work: (969) 935-0951
Fax: (969) 935-0769
Mobile: 044-999-947-5790
Email: cma_progreso@prodigy.net.mx

SURGEONS

Dr. Alvaro Quíjano
General Surgery
Address: Calle 33 #320

(corner of Calle 82)
Work: (969) 935-0951
Fax: (969) 935-0769
Mobile: 044-969-900-4610
Email: cma_progreso@prodigy.net.mx

HOSPITALS

Centro Médico Americano (C.M.A.)
Calle 33 # 320 (at the corner of Calle 82)
Notable Landmarks: Near Palacio Municipal
Colonia Centro, Progreso, Yucatán
Tel: (969) 935-0951 / 935-0769
Fax: (969) 935-0951 / 935-0769
E-mail: cma_progreso@prodigy.net.mx

PUEBLA

CARDIOLOGY

Dr. José Antonio Velasco
Internal Medicine, Cardiology, Interventional
Cardiology
Address: Calle "31 Poniente" #3327 (near Hotel
Fiesta Americana)
Borough: Colonia Las Animas
Work: (222) 249-7474, 249-8735
Fax: (222) 249-8732
Mobile: 044-222-212-6187

GASTROENTEROLOGISTS

Dr. Eduardo R. Marín
Internal Medicine, Gastroenterology,
Heptology
Address: Calle "19 Norte" #1001
Borough: Colonia Jesús García
Work: (222) 229-3700, 233-8442, ext. 1991
Fax: (222) 233-8442
Mobile: 044-222-212-4337
Pager: (222) 248-4640, PIN# 2124337
Email: e_marin@prodigy.net.mx

GYNECOLOGISTS

Dr. David Espinoza
Obstetrics & Gynecology
Address: Calle "19 Norte" #1001
Borough: Colonia Jesús García
Work: (222) 237-3509
Mobile: 044-222-954-3774
Email: despinos@prodigy.net.mx

HEPATOLOGISTS

Dr. Eduardo R. Marín
Internal Medicine, Gastroenterology,
Hepatology
Address: Calle "19 Norte" #1001
Borough: Colonia Jesús García
Work: (222) 229-3700, 233-8442, ext. 1991
Fax: (222) 233-8442
Mobile: 044-222-212-4337
Pager: (222) 248-4640, PIN# 2124337
Email: e_marin@prodigy.net.mx

INTERNIST

Dr. Eduardo R. Marín
Internal Medicine, Gastroenterology,
Hepatology
Address: Calle "19 Norte" #1001
Borough: Colonia Jesús García
Work: (222) 229-3700, 233-8442, ext. 1991
Fax: (222) 233-8442
Mobile: 044-222-212-4337
Pager: (222) 248-4640, PIN# 2124337
Email: e_marin@prodigy.net.mx

Dr. Jesús Mier
Internal Medicine, Nephrology
Address: Calle "19 Norte" #1001
Borough: Colonia Jesús García
Work: (222) 229-3700, ext. 2014 and 2013
Fax: (222) 243-6211
Mobile: 044-222-238-3525
Email: mace1123@hotmail.com.mx

Dr. José Antonio Velasco
Internal Medicine, Cardiology,
Interventional Cardiology
Address: Calle "31 Poniente" #3327 (near Hotel
Fiesta Americana)
Borough: Colonia Las Animas
Work: (222) 249-7474, 249-8735
Fax: (222) 249-8732
Mobile: 044-222-212-6187

NEPHROLOGISTS

Dr. Jesús Mier
Internal Medicine, Nephrology
Address: Calle "19 Norte" #1001
Borough: Colonia Jesús García
Work: (222) 229-3700, ext. 2014 and 2013
Fax: (222) 243-6211
Mobile: 044-222-238-3525
Email: mace1123@hotmail.com.mx

OBSTETRICIANS

Dr. David Espinoza
Obstetrics & Gynecology
Address: Calle "19 Norte" #1001
Borough: Colonia Jesús García
Work: (222) 237-3509
Mobile: 044-222-954-3774
Email: despinos@prodigy.net.mx

PEDIATRICIAN

Dr. Jesús Pulido
Pediatrics, Pediatric Intensive Care
Address: Calle "19 Norte" #1001
Borough: Colonia Jesús García
Work: (222) 231-3119, 249-3992
Fax/Home: (222) 296-1580

HOSPITALS

Hospital Español
Address: Calle "19 Norte" #1001
Main Phone #: (222) 229-3720
Fax Phone #: (222) 229-3700, ext. 1951

PUERTO AVENTURAS

EMERGENCY MEDICINE

Dr. Carlos A. Baldwin
General Medicine, Emergency Medicine
Address: house/hotel consultation only
Work: (998) 185-6543
Home: (984) 873-5494
Mobile: 044-984-801-0127
Email: docbaldwin@prodigy.net.mx

GENERAL MEDICINE

Dr. Carlos A. Baldwin
General Medicine, Emergency Medicine
Address: house/hotel consultation only
Work: (998) 185-6543
Home: (984) 873-5494
Mobile: 044-984-801-0127
Email: docbaldwin@prodigy.net.mx

Dr. Miguel Angel Galíndez
General Medicine, Homeopathy
Address: Avenida Xcacl, Lote 1
at the Hotel Catalonia
Work: (984) 875-1020, 875-5038
Home: (984) 873-5581
Mobile: 044-984-745-0486
Email: drgalindezn@hotmail.com

HOMEOPATHY

Dr. Miguel Angel Galíndez
General Medicine, Homeopathy
Address: Avenida Xcacl, Lote 1 at the
Hotel Catalonia
Work: (984) 875-1020, 875-5038
Home: (984) 873-5581
Mobile: 044-984-745-0486
Email: drgalindezn@hotmail.com

PUERTO ESCONDIDO

GENERAL MEDICINE

Dr. Maximiliano Roberto Lopez Bustamante
Ave. Oaxaca 603, Altos
Sector Juárez
Puerto Escondido, Oaxaca
Tel: (954) 582-0440

Dr. Omar Lopez Perez
Ave. Oaxaca 603, Altos
Sector Juárez
Puerto Escondido, Oaxaca
Tel: (954) 582-3634
E-mail: omarlpzprz@gmail.com

Dr. Franscisco Serrano Severiano
Blvd. del Pacifico 508
Sector Hidalgo
Puerto Escondido, Oaxaca
Tel: (954) 582-0548
Home: (954) 582-0510
Email: serranos@prodigy.net.mx

GASTROENTEROLOGISTS

Dr. José Luis Serrano
Internal Medicine, Gastroentrology
Address: Calle "10 Norte" (between
Secundaria and Conalep)
Work: (954) 582-0899
Fax: (954) 582-1278
Home: (954) 582-0203

INTERNISTS

Dr. José Luis Serrano
Internal Medicine, Gastroentrology
Address: Calle "10 Norte" (between Secundaria
and Conalep)
Work: (954) 582-0899

Fax: (954) 582-1278
Home: (954) 582-0203

HOSPITALS

Centro de Salud
Ave. Pérez Gazca 409
Colonia Centro
Puerto Escondido, Oaxaca
Tel: (954) 582-2360

Cruz Roja
7a. Norte No. 711
Colonia Centro
Puerto Escondido, Oaxaca
Tel: (954) 582-0550 / 104-2694

IMSS
2a. Poniente (no street number)
Colonia Centro
Puerto Escondido, Oaxaca
Tel: (954) 582-0349 / 0142

ISSSTE
Clínica de Especialidades y Centro de Cirugías
Simplificadas
5a. Norte and 2a. Oriente
Sector Reforma
Puerto Escondido, Oaxaca
Tel: (954) 582-1980 / 1970

Sanatorío Maria de Lourdes (Private)
Dr. Mario Cruz Ortiz
Calle Primera Poniente and Segunda Norte
Colonia Centro
Puerto Escondido, Oaxaca
Tel & Fax: (954) 582-0425 / 3859

Sanatorío San Jose (Private)
Dr. José Luis Serrano Mendez
Calle Decima Norte (no street number)
Sector Juárez
Puerto Escondido, Oaxaca
Tel: (954) 582-0899
Home: (954) 582-0203
Cell: (954) 100-4393

PUERTO PEÑASCO

GENERAL MEDICINE

Dr. Hector E. Baez Pacheco
Av. Niños Heroes y calle Benito Juarez Phone:
(638) 3-61-60

Dr. Alvaro Aburto Castro
Transmedic
Address: Juan Barrera y Nicolas Bravo
IMSS
Phone: (638) 3-27-77

Dr. José L. Contreras
Address: Corner of Símon Morúa
and Guillermo Prieto streets
Work: (638) 383-2447, 383-4040
Fax: (638) 383-5077
Home: (638) 383-1181
Mobile: 044-638-380-5312
Phone from U.S.: +1-480-704-4713
Email: clinica_santafe_@hotmail.com,
elycontreras_@hotmail.com

Dr. Francisco Landagaray
Morva y G. Prieto
Phone: (638) 3-39-04

ORTHOPEDICIANS

Dr. José Luis Olmeda
Orthopedics/Traumatology
Address: Calle Cuauhtémoc #104
(corner of Calle Lázaro Cárdenas)
Borough: Colonia Centro
Office in Puerto Penasco: (638) 383-3645
Office in Mazatlán: (669) 983-0304
Mobile: 01-669-994-7621
Email: olmedamd@hotmail.com

TRAUMATOLOGISTS

Dr. José Luis Olmeda
Orthopedics/Traumatology
Address: Calle Cuauhtémoc #104 (corner of
Calle Lázaro Cárdenas)
Borough: Colonia Centro
Office in Puerto Penasco: (638) 383-3645
Office in Mazatlán: (669) 983-0304
Mobile: 01-669-994-7621
Email: olmedamd@hotmail.com

HOSPITALS

Centro de Salud:
Simon Morua y Blvd. Juarez
Phone (638) 3-21-10

Clinica Hospital San Jose
Phone: (638) 383-1521 & 383-5121
Blvd. Benito Juarez y Gmo Prieto

Dr. Jaime Rodriguez
Clinica Santa Fe
Phone (638) 3-24-47
Simon Morua y Gmo. Prieto

Clinica Santa Maria
Niños Heroes # 37
entre Simon Morua y Serdan,
Col. Centro
Tel: 638-3832440

Dr. Alvaro Aburto Castro Transmedic
IMSS
Phone: (638) 3-27-77

Juan Barrera y Nicolas Bravo

PUERTO VALLARTA

ALLERGISTS

Dra. Ángeles Juan Pineda
Revolución 110
Conjunto Veracruz
Col. Bobadilla
Puerto Vallarta, Jalisco
Tel: (322) 224-3231
Cell Emergencies: (322) 294-0410

CARDIOLOGISTS

Dr. Jorge G. Chávez
Internal Medicine, Interventional Cardiology
Address: Calle Lucerna #148
Borough: Colonia Versalles
Work: (322) 293-1991
Fax: (322) 293-1992
Mobile: (322) 135-5500
Email: cardiomedpv@hotmail.com

Dr. Rodolfo A. Ruiz
Internal Medicine, Cardiology
Address: Calle Jesús Langarica #200-21
Borough: Colonia Centro
Work: (322) 223-0245
Fax: (322) 223-2816
Mobile: 044-322-292-1333
Pager: 01-800-723-4500, PIN# 5396040
Email: ruiznieves@yahoo.com

Dra. Leslie Swindle
Blvd. Francisco Medina Ascencio 2760-D
Zona Hotelera Norte
Puerto Vallarta, Jalisco
Tel. Amerimed: (322) 221-1088
Tel. CMQ Premiere: (322) 226-6500
Cell. Emergencies: (322) 294-0524
E-mail: swindleleslie@hotmail.com

Dr. Alejandro Valadez Jasso
Jacaranda 273
Colonia Emiliano Zapata
Puerto Vallarta, Jalisco
Tel. & Fax: (322) 222-1889
Tel. CMQ Premiere: (322) 226-6500
Cell. Emergencies: (322) 779-7738

CARDIOLOGY / CARDIOPULMONARY

Dr. Aldo Seimandi Uriarte
Clínica de Rehabilitación Cardiopulmonar y
Fisica (MedicAir)
Avenida México 993
Colonia 5 de Diciembre
Puerto Vallarta, Jalisco
Tel.: (322) 222-1596
Fax: (322) 222-1699
E-mail: medicair@prodigy.net.mx

COLPOSCOPY

Dr. Armando Ortiz
Obstetrics & Gynecology, Colposcopy
Address: Calle Cenzontle #102
Borough: Colonia Las Aralias
Work/Fax: (322) 225-5023
Mobile: 044-322-294-1347
Email: aortiza_mx@hotmail.com

DENTISTS

Dental Center
Dra. Carla Iliana Rangel
Dr. Fernando Mendoza
Calle Yugoslavia 149
Col. Versalles
Puerto Vallarta, Jalisco
Tel.: (322) 224-5585 / 225-4225
Cell Emergencies: (322) 294-0588

Grupo Odontologico Integral
Dra. Leticia Armas Tejeda
Plaza Marina, Local G24 - G25

Carretera Aeropuerto Km 8
Marina Vallarta
Puerto Vallarta , Jalisco
Tel.: (322) 221-2215
Cell. Emergencies: (322) 100-8691 / (
322) 728-0564
Website: www.dentalofficepuertovallarta.com

Unident
Condominios Royal Pacific
Calle Timón (no street number), Local D
Marina Vallarta
Puerto Vallarta, Jalisco
Tel.: (322) 209-0099 / 0999
E-mail: blvalle@hotmail.com
Website: www.dentistvallarta.com

DERMATOLOGISTS

Dr. Eduardo Cervantes Gutiérrez
Clínica Integral
Ave. Los Tules 146
Col. Díaz Ordaz
Puerto Vallarta, Jalisco
Tel. & Fax: (322) 293-6090
Cell. Emergencies: (322) 306-0465
E-mail: ecerv@prodigy.net.mx

Dra. Mariza Tamayo Rodriguez
Lucerna 145
Col. Versalles
Puerto Vallarta, Jalisco
Tel.: (322) 224-9898 / 9292
Cell. Emergencies: (33) 1169-6467
E-mail: dermariza@hotmail.com

EAR, NOSE & THROAT

Dr. Luciano Aguirre Mora
CMQ Hospital
Basilio Badillo 365
Colonia Emiliano Zapata
Puerto Vallarta, Jalisco
Tel.: (322) 223-1919 / 223-0011

Dr. Jorge Maciel Bejar
Manuel M. Dieguez 358-A

Col. Emiliano Zapata
Puerto Vallarta, Jalisco
Tel. & Fax: (322) 223-0444
Cell. Emergencies: (322) 294-9865

FAMILY DOCTORS

Dr. Peter Gordon
Avenida Los Tules 116, Int 14
Colonia Diaz Ordaz
Puerto Vallarta, Jalisco
Tel: (322) 293-1552 / 1553 / 225-3440
E-mail: pgordonmd@gmail.com

GENERAL MEDICINE

Dr. Luis G. Arias
General Medicine
Address: Calle Lucerna #148
Borough: Colonia Versalles
Work: (322) 293-1991
Fax: (322) 293-1992
Mobile: 044-322-779-8000
Email: dr.arias@mail.com

Dr. César Enrique Cerda Acuña
Dra. Linda Noemi Betancourt Quintero
Dr. Pedro Parada González
(Hotel calls & visits)
CMQ Premiere Hospital
Francisco Villa 1749
Colonia Vallarta Villas,
Puerto Vallarta, Jalisco
Tel: (322) 226 6500
Cell Phones:
Dr. César Enrique Cerda Acuña:
(322) 182-1280
Dra. Linda Noemi Betancourt Quintero:
(322) 147-6735
Dr. Pedro Parada Gonzalez:
(322) 117-8765

GYNECOLOGISTS

Dr. Humberto Aguirre
Plaza Comercial Puerto Iguana Local 2

Puerto Vallarta, Jalisco
Tel. & Fax: (322) 221-2771
Cell. Emergencies: (322) 294-0727
E-mail: doctorhaguirre@hotmail.com

Dra. Laura García
Jacarandas 273
Col. Emiliano Zapata
Puerto Vallarta, Jalisco
Tel.: (322) 222-1889
Cell. Emergencies: (322) 779-7739
E-mail: laurachina@yahoo.com

Dr. Jorge Hernández Amaya
Hospital Cornerstone
Av. Los Tules 136, 1er piso
Colonia Diaz Ordaz
Puerto Vallarta, Jalisco
Tel.: (322) 223 2246

Dr. Armando Ortiz
Obstetrics & Gynecology, Colposcopy
Address: Calle Cenzontle #102
Borough: Colonia Las Aralias
Work/Fax: (322) 225-5023
Mobile: 044-322-294-1347
Email: aortiza_mx@hotmail.com

INTENSIVE CARE

Dr. Alejandro Ríos
Internal Medicine, Pulmonology,
Intensive Care
Address: Boulevard Francisco Medina
Ascencio #2760
Work: (322) 293-0529
Fax: (322) 226-1010
Home: (322) 209-0413
Mobile: 044-322-779-7118
Email: arios@sanjaviermarina.com

INTERNISTS

Dr. Jorge G. Chávez
Internal Medicine, Interventional Cardiology
Address: Calle Lucerna #148
Borough: Colonia Versalles

Work: (322) 293-1991
Fax: (322) 293-1992
Mobile: (322) 135-5500
Email: cardiomedpv@hotmail.com

Dr. Aldo Curiel
Internal Medicine, Nephrology
Address: Calle Lucerna #148
Borough: Colonia Versalles
Work: (322) 293-1991
Fax: (322) 223-8007
Mobile: 044-322-294-1797
Pager: 01-800-527-7979, PIN# 5689183
Email: drcuriel@hotmail.com

Dr. Antonio Matilla
(Hotel calls and visits)
Address: Boulevard Francisco Medina
Ascencio, Plaza Neptuno, F-4,
Marina Vallarta (near the Marina Golf course)
Tel: (322) 226-6500, (322) 221-1088,
226-2080
Home: (322) 297-1508
Cell for Emergencies: (322) 294-1631
E-mail: matillaa@hotmail.com
24 hours service

Dr. Alejandro Ríos
Internal Medicine, Pulmonology,
Intensive Care
Address: Boulevard Francisco Medina Ascencio
#2760
Work: (322) 293-0529
Fax: (322) 226-1010
Home: (322) 209-0413
Mobile: 044-322-779-7118
Email: arios@sanjaviermarina.com

Dr. Rodolfo A. Ruiz
Internal Medicine, Cardiology
Address: Calle Jesús Langarica #200-21
Borough: Colonia Centro
Work: (322) 223-0245
Fax: (322) 223-2816
Mobile: 044-322-292-1333
Pager: 01-800-723-4500, PIN# 5396040
Email: ruiznieves@yahoo.com

Dra. Leslie Ann Swindle
Internal Medicine, Cardiology, Nuclear
Cardiology
Address: Boulevard Francisco Medina
Ascencio, Plaza Neptuno, F-4,
Marina Vallarta (near the Marina Golf course)
Work: (322) 221-1088
Mobile: 044-322-294-0524
Email: swindleleslie@hotmail.com

NATURAL MEDICINE

Dr. Nelson Sánchez Soto
Calle Yugoslavia 149
Colonia Versalles
Puerto Vallarta, Jalisco
Tel.: (322) 225-4225
(Spanish only)

NEPHROLOGISTS

Dr. Aldo Curiel
Internal Medicine, Nephrology
Address: Calle Lucerna #148
Borough: Colonia Versalles
Work: (322) 293-1991
Fax: (322) 223-8007
Mobile: 044-322-294-1797
Pager: 01-800-527-7979, PIN# 5689183
Email: drcuriel@hotmail.com

NEUROLOGISTS

Dr. Javier Aguilar Lopez
Francisco Villa 880
Col. Las Gaviotas
Puerto Vallarta, Jalisco
Tel.: (322) 225-6008
Home: (322) 225-6785
Cell. Emergencies: (322) 292-1735
(Spanish only)

OBSTETRICIANS

Dr. Armando Ortiz
Obstetrics & Gynecology, Colposcopy
Address: Calle Cenzontle #102
Borough: Colonia Las Aralias
Work/Fax: (322) 225-5023
Mobile: 044-322-294-1347
Email: aortiza_mx@hotmail.com

OPHTHALMOLOGISTS

Dra. Mónica Gómez Rosenzweig
Paraguay 1092
Colonia 5 de Diciembre
Puerto Vallarta, Jalisco
Tel.: (322) 222-0019

Dr. Jaime Miramontes Contreras
CMQ Premiere
Francisco Villa 1749
Col. Vallarta Villas
Puerto Vallarta, Jalisco
Tel.: (322) 226-6500
Cell. Emergencies: (322) 205-7116
Fax: (322) 223-1919
E-mail: drjmiramontes@hotmail.com

ORTHOPEDISTS

Dr. Max Greig
Orthopedics/Traumatology, Sports Medicine
Address: Avenida Los Tules #136
(next to Plaza Caracol)
Borough: Colonia Díaz Ordaz
Work: (322) 224-9400, ext. 137
Fax: (322) 293-1992
Home: (322) 222-3627
Mobile: 044-322-205-7117
Email: maxgreig@yahoo.com

Dr. Jorge Martínez Garza
Orthopedics/Traumatology, Pediatric
Orthopedic Surgery
Address: Avenida Francisco Medina
Ascencio #2760
Borough: Colonia Zona Hotelera Norte

Office hours: M–F: 10am–2pm,
Work/Fax: (322) 226-1010
Mobile: 044-322-306-0013
Email: jmtzgf@hotmail.com

Dr. Luis Fernando Villanueva
CMQ Hospital
Basilio Badillo 365
Col. Emiliano Zapata
Puerto Vallarta, Jalisco
Tel.: (322) 223-6011 / 222-5119
Emergencies: (322) 223-1919

PEDIATRICIANS

Dra. María L. Aréchiga
Pediatrics
Address: Avenida Los Tules #136,
Office 201 (next to Plaza Caracol)
Borough: Colonia Díaz Ordaz
Work/Fax: (322) 293-3601
Mobile: 044-322-429-7773
Email: doctora_leticia@hotmail.com

Dr. Fernando Diaz Otero
CMQ Premiere
Francisco Villa 1749
Colonia Fovissste, Puerto Vallarta, Jalisco
Tel.: (322) 226-6500

Dr. Salvador González Navarro
CMQ Premiere
Francisco Villa 1749
Colonia Fovissste
Puerto Vallarta, Jalisco
Tel.: (322) 226-6500

Dr. Antonio Mota
Alameda 603
Colonia El Calvario
Puerto Vallarta, Jalisco
Tel.: (322) 225-9048
Cell. Emergencies: (322) 227-2695

Dr. Jesús Ochoa Vargas
CMQ Premiere
Francisco Villa 1749
Colonia Fovissste

Puerto Vallarta, Jalisco
Tel.: (322) 226-6500
Cell. Emergencies: (322) 294-2507
E-mail: drjeova68@hotmail.com
(Spanish only)

PEDIATRIC ORTHOPEDIC SURGERY

Dr. Jorge Martínez Garza
Orthopedics/Traumatology, Pediatric
Orthopedic Surgery
Address: Avenida Francisco Medina
Ascencio #2760
Borough: Colonia Zona Hotelera Norte
Office hours: M–F: 10am–2pm,
Work/Fax: (322) 226-1010
Mobile: 044-322-306-0013
Email: jmtzgf@hotmail.com

PLASTIC SURGEONS

Dr. Alejandro Guerrero
CMQ Premiere Hospital
Francisco Villa 1749
Colonia Fovissste, Puerto Vallarta, Jalisco
Tel.: (322) 226-6500

Dr. Ricardo Rivera García
Clínica Intermédica
Lucerna 148
Colonia Versalles, Puerto Vallarta, Jalisco
Tel. & Fax: (322) 293-1991
Cell. Emergencies: (33) 1036-5191
E-mail: drriveragarcia@telcel.blackberry.net;
arquiplastics@prodigy.net.mx

PSYCHIATRISTS

Dra. Adi Janette Dominguez De Alba
Médica Fluvial
Lago Tangañica 222
at corner with Río Santiago
Fluvial Vallarta
Puerto Vallarta, Jalisco

Tel.: (322) 225-8787 / 223-6387
E-mail: psicogeriatra@gmail.com

Dr. Enrique Sinencio Herrera
Rafael Osuna 120, corner with Berlin
Colonia Versalles
Puerto Vallarta, Jalisco
Tel.: (322) 225-6262
Cell. Emergencies only: (322) 100-1364
E-mail: esinencio@hotmail.com

PULMONOLOGY

Dr. Alejandro Ríos
Internal Medicine, Pulmonology,
Intensive Care
Address: Boulevard Francisco Medina
Ascencio #2760
Work: (322) 293-0529
Fax: (322) 226-1010
Home: (322) 209-0413
Mobile: 044-322-779-7118
Email: arios@sanjaviermarina.com

RADIOLOGISTS

Centro de Imagenología &
Laboratorios Vallarta
Ave. Los Tules 152
Col. Díaz Ordaz
Puerto Vallarta, Jalisco
Tel.: (322) 224-4287 / 293-7321

Dra. Cynthia Lorena Cortez
CMQ Premiere
Francisco Villa 1749
Col. Fovissste
Puerto Vallarta, Jalisco
Tel.: (322) 226-6500
Cell. Emergencies: (322) 108-9139

REHABILITATION

Lizaola Rehabilitation Center
Fluvial Vallarta 267
Col. Fluvial Vallarta
Puerto Vallarta, Jalisco
Tel.: (322) 224-7997

SPORTS MEDICINE

Dr. Max Greig
Orthopedics/Traumatology, Sports Medicine
Address: Avenida Los Tules #136
(next to Plaza Caracol)
Borough: Colonia Díaz Ordaz
Work: (322) 224-9400, ext. 137
Fax: (322) 293-1992
Home: (322) 222-3627
Mobile: 044-322-205-7117
Email: maxgreig@yahoo.com

SURGEONS

Dr. José Luis Bernal Martinez
CMQ Premiere
Francisco Villa 1749
Colonia Fovissste
Puerto Vallarta, Jalisco
Tel. & Fax: (322) 226-6500
Emergencies: (322) 293-8823

Dr. Rafael Lujan Rodríguez
CMQ Hospital
Basilio Badillo 365
Col. Emiliano Zapata
Puerto Vallarta, Jalisco
Tel.: (322) 223-0011 / 222-5119
Fax: (322) 223-1919
Cell. Emergencies: (322) 105-0256

TRAUMATOLOGISTS

Dr. Max Greig
Orthopedics/Traumatology, Sports Medicine
Address: Avenida Los Tules #136
(next to Plaza Caracol)
Borough: Colonia Díaz Ordaz
Work: (322) 224-9400, ext. 137
Fax: (322) 293-1992
Home: (322) 222-3627
Mobile: 044-322-205-7117
Email: maxgreig@yahoo.com

Dr. Jorge Martínez Garza
Orthopedics/Traumatology, Pediatric

Orthopedic Surgery
Address: Avenida Francisco Medina
Ascencio #2760
Borough: Colonia Zona Hotelera Norte
Work/Fax: (322) 226-1010
Mobile: 044-322-306-0013
Email: jmtzgf@hotmail.com
Office hours: M–F: 10am–2pm,

UROLOGISTS

Dr. Pedro López
Urologist
Address: Avenida Los Tules #136,
Office 203
Borough: Colonia Díaz Ordaz
Office: (322) 225-1183
Mobile: 044-322-779-7154
Email: lopezcroto@hotmail.com

AMBULANCES

CMQ AMBULANCE
CMQ Premiere Hospital
Francisco Villa 1749
Colonia Fovissste
Puerto Vallarta, Jalisco
Tel.: (322) 226 6500
E-mail: cmqpremiere@gmail.com

Cruz Roja
Río Balsas y Río Plata
Col. López Mateos
Puerto Vallarta, Jalisco
Tel.: (322) 222-1533
Fax: (322) 222-4973
(Only Spanish spoken)

Mexico Accessible
(Wheelchairs and Ground Transportation)
Océano Indico 399
Colonia Palmar de Aramara
Puerto Vallarta, Jalisco
Tel.: (322) 225 0989 / 224 1868
Email: info@accessiblemexico.com
Website: www.accesiblemexico.com

HOSPITALS - PRIVATE

AmeriMed-Puerto Vallarta
Address: Boulevard Francisco Medina Ascencio, Plaza Neptuno, Suite D-1
Borough: Marina Vallarta
Notable Landmarks: Near the bull ring, 2 kms from the airport
Main Phone #: (322) 226-2080
Fax Phone #: (322) 226-2060

CMQ
Basilio Badillo 365
Col. Emiliano Zapata
Puerto Vallarta, Jalisco
Tel. & Fax: (322) 223-1919/2423

CMQ Premiere
Francisco Villa 1749
Col. Fovissste
Puerto Vallarta, Jalisco
Tel. & Fax: (322) 226-6500

Hospital Cornerstone
Address: Avenida Los Tules #136
Borough: Colonia Diaz Ordaz
Landmarks: One block from Plaza Caracol
Main/Fax Phone #: (322) 224-9400, ext. 137
Website: www.hospitalcornerstone.com

Hospital San Javier Marina
Address: Boulevard Francisco Medina
Ascencio #2760
Borough: Zona Hotelera Norte
Notable Landmarks: Near Gas Station
de Terminal Marítima
Main Phone #: (322) 226-1000, 226-1010, 226-1013, 226-1014, 226-1015
Fax Phone #: (322) 226-1010

HOSPITALS - PUBLIC

Cruz Roja
Río Balsas y Río Plata
Col. López Mateos
Puerto Vallarta, Jalisco
Tel.: (322) 222-1533

Fax: (322) 222-4973
(Only Spanish spoken)

Regional
Calle Dinamarca esq. Noruega
Col. Villas del Real
Puerto Vallarta, Jalisco
Tel.: (322) 299-5600/5601/5603
(Only Spanish spoken)

QUERETARO

CARDIOLOGISTS

Dr. Eliodoro Castro
Internal Medicine, Cardiology
Address: Calle Bernardino del Razo #21
Borough: Colonia Ensueño
Work: (442) 192-3077
Fax: (442) 192-3076
Mobile: 044-442-226-2544
Email: elidoroc@prodigy.net.mx

Dr. Salvador León
Internal Medicine, Cardiology
Address: Calle Bernardino del Razo #21,
Office 135-B
Work/Fax: (442) 192-3042
Heart Institute: (442) 216-2745
Mobile: 044-442-186-0404
Email: leons@prodigy.net.mx

DIABETES

Dr. Manuel Bañales
Internal Medicine, Diabetes
Address: Calle Bernardino del Razo #21,
Office 135
Borough: Colonia Ensueño
Work: (442) 192-3041, 192-3042, 192-3043
Fax: (442) 192-3041
Mobile: 044-442-190-3198

Home: (442) 213-9235
Email: drham1@hotmail.com

GYNECOLOGISTS

Dra. Mercedes Birlain
Obstetrics & Gynecology, Laparoscopy
Address: Calle Bernardino del Razo #21,
Office 335
Work: (442) 216-5118, 192-3092
Fax: (442) 192-3092
Mobile: 044-442-190-3080
Email: mbirlain@hotmail.com

INTERNISTS

Dr. Manuel Bañales
Internal Medicine, Diabetes
Address: Calle Bernardino del Razo #21,
Office 135
Borough: Colonia Ensueño
Work: (442) 192-3041, 192-3042, 192-3043
Fax: (442) 192-3041
Mobile: 044-442-190-3198
Home: (442) 213-9235
Email: drham1@hotmail.com

Dr. Eliodoro Castro
Internal Medicine, Cardiology
Address: Calle Bernardino del Razo #21
Borough: Colonia Ensueño
Work: (442) 192-3077
Fax: (442) 192-3076
Mobile: 044-442-226-2544
Email: elidoroc@prodigy.net.mx

Dr. Salvador León
Internal Medicine, Cardiology
Address: Calle Bernardino del Razo #21,
Office 135-B
Work/Fax: (442) 192-3042
Heart Institute: (442) 216-2745
Mobile: 044-442-186-0404
Email: leons@prodigy.net.mx

LAPARASCOPY

Dra. Mercedes Birlain
Obstetrics & Gynecology, Laparoscopy
Address: Calle Bernardino del Razo #21,
Office 335
Work: (442) 216-5118, 192-3092
Fax: (442) 192-3092
Mobile: 044-442-190-3080
Email: mbirlain@hotmail.com

OBSTETRICIAN

Dra. Mercedes Birlain
Obstetrics & Gynecology, Laparoscopy
Address: Calle Bernardino del Razo #21,
Office 335
Work: (442) 216-5118, 192-3092
Fax: (442) 192-3092
Mobile: 044-442-190-3080
Email: mbirlain@hotmail.com

ORTHOPEDICIANS

Dr. Fidel G. Dobarganes
Orthopedics/Traumatology
Address: Libramiento a Dolores
Hidalgo #43, Suite 2
Borough: Colonia Mesa del Malanquín
Work: (415) 152-2233
Fax: (442) 192-3083
Mobile: (442) 281-0981
Pager: 01-800-723-4500, PIN#: 1488
Nextel: 014421253578
Email: fdobarganes@prodigy.net.mx

TRAUMATOLOGISTS

Dr. Fidel G. Dobarganes
Orthopedics/Traumatology
Address: Libramiento a Dolores
Hidalgo #43, Suite 2
Borough: Colonia Mesa del Malanquín
Work: (415) 152-2233
Fax: (442) 192-3083

Mobile: (442) 281-0981
Pager: 01-800-723-4500, PIN#: 1488
Nextel: 014421253578
Email: fdobarganes@prodigy.net.mx

HOSPITALS

Hospital Angeles de Querétaro
Address: Calle Bernardino del Razo #21
Borough: Colonia Ensueño
Notable Landmarks: A few blocks from
the Querétaro – Celaya libre freeway
Main Phone #: (442) 192-3000
Fax Phone #: (442) 192-3095
Emergency Phone #: (442) 215-5901

Hospital San José de Querétaro
Address: Prolongación Constituyentes
(at the corner of Calle Hacienda Santillán)
Borough: Fraccionamiento Jacal
Main Phone #: (442) 211-0080
Fax Phone #: (442) 211-0080, ext. 2282
Emergency Phone #: (442) 211-0080, ext.
2294, 2296

REYNOSA

DENTISTS

Dra. Patricia García Chacon,
Specializing in: Integral Odontology
Calle Morelos Pte. # 125, Zona Centro
Office hours: 9 am to 1 pm & from
3 pm to 8 pm Monday–Friday
Tel & Fax: (899) 9 22 45 45
E-mail: patriciagarciach@hotmail.com
Universidad Autónoma de Nuevo León
Thirty-years of experience

Dr. Américo López Garza,
Specializing in: Integral Odontology
Morelos Poniente No. 125, Zona Centro

Office hours: 9 am to 1 pm & from
3 pm to 8 pm Monday–Friday
Tel & Fax: (899) 9 22 45 45
Universidad Autónoma de Nuevo León
Forty-eight years of experience.

INTERNISTS

Dr. Francisco Cano García,
Pedro José Mendez No. 100,
Colonia Del Prado
Office hours: 10 am to 7 pm Monday–Friday
Tel: (899) 9 22 22 60
Fax: (899) 9 22 37 49
E-mail: mdfco_cano@hotmail.com
Universidad Autónoma de Nuevo León & Hospital Dr. Jose Eleuterio González in Nuevo León
Twenty-five years of experience.

NEUROLOGISTS

Dr. Héctor Serrano Martínez,
Specializing in: Neurology & Neurosurgery
Calle Guadalupe Victoria #994, Zona Centro
Office hours: 9 am to 1 pm & from
4 pm to 6 pm Monday–Friday
Tel & Fax: (899) 9 22 43 95
E-mail: serranar3910@hotmail.com
Universidad Veracruzana, Universidad
Nacional Autonoma de México, Hospital
20 de Noviembre, México, D.F. and
Hospital Juarez
Thirty-three years of experience.

PEDIATRICIANS

Dr. José Gabriel Rosado Triay,
Calle Ortíz Rubio No. 531,
Colonia del Prado
Office hours: 9:30 am to 12:30 pm &
from 5 pm to 7 pm Monday–Friday
Tel: (899) 9 22 05 36
Fax: (899) 9 22 33 60
E-mail: jrosado@hotmail.com
Universidad Nacional Autónoma de México

& Hospital 20 de Noviembre, Mexico City.
Twenty-eight years of experience.

HOSPITALS

Centro de Salud
Boulevard Morelos y Toluca
(no street number), Col. Rodríguez
Tel: (899) 925 05 60, 923 79 36

Clinica-Hospital Victoria
Guadalupe Victoria # 826, Zona Centro
Tel: (899) 9 22 90 51, 9 22 90 41
Fax: (899) 9 22 86 50 11

Hospital Christus Muguerza
La Ribereña, km 5.5
Tel: (899) 909-69 00, 909 69 63, 909 69 51
E-mail: cmr@christusmuguerza.com.mx
http://www.christusmuguerza.com.mx/hospital-reynosa/

Hospital de Especialidaes Santander
P. Ortiz Rubio y Francisco I. Madero,
Col. Del Prado.
Tel: (899) 9 21 67 00

Hospital Esperanza
Veracruz # 542 Ote.
Colonia Rodríguez
Tel: (899) 9 22 77 10, 9 22 77 15,
9 22 52 11, 9 22 52 87

Hospital Las Fuentes
Blvd. Del Maestro # 530
Col. Las Fuentes
Tel: (899) 9 25 50 22, 9 25 50 23, 9 25 53 85

Hospital Regional del Rio
Libramiento Echeverría y Río Bravo,
Colonia Del Prado
Tel: (899) 9 22 52 01, 9 22 51 02
Fax: (899) 9 22 50 87

Hospital Tierra Santa
Blvd. Inglaterra # 135, Esq. Con Flores Magón,
Colonia Canadá
Tel: (899) 9 24 28 22, 9 23 78 80

SALTILLO

GENERAL MEDICINE

Dr. Jorge Eduardo Mellado
Blvd. Venustiano Carranza 4036
Colonia Virreyes Residencial
Saltillo, Coahuila
Tel: (844) 416-1022 / 9992
Evenings only

PSYCHOLOGISTS

Dr. Javier Cárdena
Dra. Alicia Casanueva
Rufino Tamayo 100
Fraccionamiento San Isidro
Saltillo, Coahuila
Tel: (844) 415-1191

HOSPITALS

Cruz Roja
Presidente Cárdenas y Rayón
Colonia Saltillo, Zona Centro
Saltillo, Coahuila
Tel: (844) 414-3333

Centro Hospitalario La Concepción
Blvd. Venustiano Carranza #4036,
Col. Virreyes Residencial
Saltillo, Coahuila de Zaragoza,
Telephone (844) 450-6000 & 416-1022

Hospital Cheristus Maguerza
Carretera Monterrey-Saltillo Km. 4.5
Saltillo, Coahuila
Tel: (844) 411-7000
Fax (844) 411-7060

Hospital Concepcion
Venustiano Carranza Norte 4036
Colonia Villa Olímpica

Saltillo, Coahuila
Tel: (844) 416-1022

Hospital Magisterio
Boulevard Antonio Cárdenas
(no street number)
Colonia Ferrocarrileros
Saltillo, Coahuila
Tel: (844) 417-3062

Hospital Universitario de Saltillo
Calzada Francisco I. Madero #1291,
Zona Centro
Saltillo, Coahuila de Zaragoza,
Telephone (844) 411-3000 al 05
Fax (844) 412-7935

SAN CARLOS, NUEVO GUAYMAS

GENERAL MEDICINE

Dr. José Luis Canale
General Medicine, Gerontology
Address: Calle Marte, Lot 96
Town: San Carlos
Work/Fax: (662) 226-0062
Mobile: (662) 044-622-855-9954
Email: joseluisdoc@yahoo.com

CARDIOLOGY

Dr. Horacio E. Erausquin
Plaza los Jitos local 30 Internal Medicine
San Carlos, N. Guaymas, Sonora,
Phone: (622) 226-1585
Email: eurasquin@prodigy.net.mx
Hours: 9 AM to 12 AM,
Mondays, Wednesdays and Fridays only.

FAMILY MEDICINE

Dr. José Luis Canale Escalante
Lote 96 Calle Marte, El Creston
San Carlos, N. Guaymas, Sonora
Tel. & Fax: (622) 226-0062
E-mail: joseluisdoc@yahoo.com
info@clinicasancarlos.com
www.clinicasancarlos.com

GERONTOLOGISTS

Dr. José Luis Canale
General Medicine, Gerontology
Address: Calle Marte, Lot 96
Town: San Carlos
Work/Fax: (662) 226-0062
Mobile: (662) 044-622-855-9954
Email: joseluisdoc@yahoo.com

HOSPITALS

Clínica San Carlos
Address: Calle Marte Lot 96
Borough: El Creston, San Carlos
Notable Landmarks: Across from Banamex
Bank and PEMEX station
Main/Fax Phone #: (622) 226-0062
(request fax tone)
Website: www.cscsancarlos.com

SAN CRISTOBAL DE LAS CASAS

GENERAL PRACTITIONERS

Dr. Raymundo Albaran Carbajal
Ave. Benito Juárez 34-B
Barrio de Santa Lucia
San Cristóbal de las Casas, Chiapas

Tel: (967) 116-0685
Emergencies: (967) 127-5151 / 119-2539
E-mail: ygyamauchi@yahoo.com.mx

Dr. Luis José R. Sevilla
General Medicine
Address: Calle de Sol #12
Borough: Colonia Bizmark
Work: (967) 678-1626
Mobile: 044-967-677-5672

Dr. Renato Zarate
General Medicine, Parasitic Medicine
Address: Avenida Juárez #60
Borough: Colonia Santa Lucia
Work: (967) 678-0793, 678-2294
Home: (967) 678-2998
Mobile: 044-967-101-1362
Email: zarategreengreen@prodigy.net.mx

PARASITIC MEDICINE

Dr. Renato Zarate
General Medicine, Parasitic Medicine
Address: Avenida Juárez #60
Borough: Colonia Santa Lucia
Work: (967) 678-0793, 678-2294
Home: (967) 678-2998
Mobile: 044-967-101-1362
Email: zarategreengreen@prodigy.net.mx

HOSPITALS

Centro de Salud
1a. Calle de los Pinos (no street number)
Barrio de los Pinos
San Cristóbal de las Casas,
Chiapas
Tel: (967) 678-0609

Cruz Roja
Ave. Ignacio Allende No. 57
Colonia Altejar
San Cristóbal de las Casas, Chiapas
Tel: (967) 678-0772 / 6565

Hospital General
Insurgentes 24
Barrio de Santa Lucia
San Cristóbal de las Casas,
Chiapas
Tel: (967) 678-0770 / 678-3834

SAN FELIPE

GENERAL MEDICINE

Dr. Victor Abasolo
Calzada Chetumal, no street number
(½ block from the 7-11 convenience store)
Tel/Fax: (686) 577-1706
Home: (686) 577-1458
Cel: 044-686-573-0174
e-mail: victorchela@direcway.com

GYNECOLOGISTS

Dr. Gerardo Arano
Avenida Mar Negro #1285
Tel: (686) 577-0117, 577-2976
Fax: (686) 577-2849
Cel: 044-686-569-2874
Home: (686) 566-2045

OBSTETRICIANS

Dr. Gerardo Arano
Avenida Mar Negro #1285
Tel: (686) 577-0117, 577-2976
Fax: (686) 577-2849
Cel: 044-686-569-2874
Home: (686) 566-2045

HOSPITALS

Hospital San Felipe
Avenida Mar Negro #1285

Central region
Notable Landmarks: Next to police
department
Tel: (686) 577-0117
Fax: (686) 577-2849

SAN FERNANDO

CARDIOLOGISTS

Dr. Rodolfo Chible A. González,
Carretera Victoria-Matamoros No. 412
Office hours: 10 am to 3 pm &
5 pm to 9 pm Monday–Friday
Tel: (841) 84 4 02 56
Fax: (841) 84 4 11 30
E-mail: rchible@prodigy.net.mx
Universidad Autónoma de México and
Centro Médico Nacional
Twenty-seven years of experience.

GENERAL MEDICINE

Dr. Jesús Francisco Aranda Zamarripa,
Carretera Victoria-Matamoros#412,
entre Ruíz Cortinez y Terán
Office hours: 8 am to 8 pm
Tel: (841) 844-0256
E-mail: dr.jfarandax@hotmail.com
Facultad de Ciencias de la Salud de la Univer-
sidad Autónoma de Tamaulipas
Six years of experience.

Dr. Gabriel Angel Martínez De La Garza
Calle Bravo y Juarez #509,
Zona Centro
Office hours: 5 pm to 9 pm
Tel: (841) 844-02 56
E-mail: dr.gabrielmtz@gmail.com
Universidad de Monterrey
Seventheen years of experience.

HOSPITALS

Centro de Salud
Calle Porfirio Díaz y Cristobal Colón
(no street number),
Colonia Loma Alta
Tel: (841) 852-3498 and
(841) 844-1750 15

Hospital General
Carretera Victoria-Matamoros km. 173
Tel: (841) 844-04 94, 04 95.

SAN JOSE DEL CABO
(ALSO SEE CABO SAN LUCAS)

AMBULANCES

Medcare Ambulance Services
(Admninistrative Offices)
Carretera Transpeninsular Km.1
Col. Magisterial
San José del Cabo,
Baja California Sur
Tel: (624) 142-5255
Offices in San Felipe:
Tel: (686) 57 70500

CARDIOLOGISTS

Dr. Alejandro Valderráin Zazueta
Paseo Marinos (entre Pescador y Barco)
Col. Chamizal, San José del Cabo,
Baja California Sur
Tel: (624) 142-1994 / 3031
Cell: (624) 122-0456

DENTISTS

Dr. Romeo Gamboa Castañares
Plaza California 11, 2nd. Floor
San José del Cabo,
Baja California Sur

Tel: (624) 142-2581
Fax: (624) 142-4745
E-mail: drgamboa@prodigy.net.mx

Dr. Jose Antonio Garcia Montemayor
Benito Juarez 1717, local 1
Col. Centro, San Jose del Cabo
Tel: 624 1469625
Cell 6243553030

GENERAL MEDICINE

Dr. Javier Palacios
Address: Transpeninsular Highway, km 28,
Plaza El Zalate, Local 3
Borough: Colonia Costa Azul
City: San José del Cabo
Work/Fax: (624) 130-7011
Mobile: 044-624-145-2360
Email: palaciossj@hotmail.com

GERIATRICIAN

Dr. Alfonso Jurado
Address: Transpeninsular Highway, km 28,
Plaza El Zalate, Local 3
Borough: Colonia Costa Azul
City: San José del Cabo
Work/Fax: (624) 130-7011
Mobile: 044-624-147-5881
Email: alfonsojuradomd@yahoo.com

INTERNIST

Dr. Alfonso Jurado
Address: Transpeninsular Highway, km 28,
Plaza El Zalate, Local 3
Borough: Colonia Costa Azul
City: San José del Cabo
Work/Fax: (624) 130-7011
Mobile: 044-624-147-5881
Email: alfonsojuradomd@yahoo.com

OBSTETRICIANS/ GYNECOLOGISTS

Dra. María Elena Valderráin Zazueta
Paseo Marinos (entre Pescador y Barco)
Col. Chamizal, San José del Cabo,
Baja California Sur
Tel: (624) 142-1994 / 3031
Cell: (624) 122-1585

ORTHOPEDISTS

Dr. José Pablo Arriaga Lizárraga
Paseo Marinos (near the corner of Barco), 2nd
Floor
Col. Chamizal, San José del Cabo,
Baja California Sur
Tel: (624) 142-6565
Cell: (624) 145-2621

PEDIATRICIANS

Dr. Enrique Gutiérrez Garro
Marina (between Pescador and Barco),
Local 3
Col. Chamizal, San José del Cabo,
Baja California Sur
Tel: (624) 142-2711
Cell: (624) 142-2599

Dr. Gildardo Rodriguez
Paseo Marinos and Pescador
Col. Chamizal, San José del Cabo,
Baja California Sur
Tel: (624) 142-2411
Cell: (624) 140-1252
Emergencies: (624) 142-2883

RADIOLOGISTS

Dr. Aníbal H. Hernández
Zaragoza 13
Colonia San José del Cabo
San José del Cabo,
Baja California Sur
Tel: (624) 142-1203

SURGEONS

Dr. José Pablo Arriaga Lizárraga
Paseo Marinos (near the corner of Barco),
2nd Floor
Col. Chamizal, San José del Cabo,
Baja California Sur
Tel: (624) 142-6565
Cell: (624) 145-2621

Dr. Jorge Holguín Aragón
Marina (between Pescador and Barco),
Local 3
Col. Chamizal, San José del Cabo,
Baja California Sur
Tel: (624) 142-2711
Cell: (624) 145-2957

HOSPITALS

Amerimed Hospital
Plaza Cabo Ley
Paseo de las Misiones (no street number),
Locales 1 and 2
Col. Campo de Golf
San José del Cabo,
Baja California Sur
Tel: (624) 105-8550
Fax: (624) 142-2880

Clínica San José
Marinos, esq. Barco y Panga
Col. Chamizal, San José del Cabo,
Baja California Sur
Tel: (624) 142-0260
Fax: (624) 142-3257

Cruz Roja
Boulevard Mijares (no street number)
Colonia Centro
San José del Cabo,
Baja California Sur
Tel: (624) 142-0316
Fax: (624) 142-2188

Hospital General
Marinos (no street number)
Col. Chamizal, San José del Cabo,
Baja California Sur
Tel: (624) 142-3813 / 0013

SAN LUIS POTOSI

CARDIOLOGY

Dr. José Luis Arenas-León
Internal Medicine, Cardiology
Address: Calle Antonio Aguilar #155,
Office V-4
Borough: Colonia Burócratas del Estado
Work: (444) 817-7013
Mobile: 044-444-803-7057
Pager: (444) 812-7766, PIN #1015291
Email: jlarenas@saludangeles.com

CARDIOPULMONARY MEDICINE

Dr. Alejandro Quesada
Internal Medicine, Cardiopulmonary Medicine
Address: Calle Madre Perla #435,
Office 217
Borough: Fraccionamiento Indústrias
Work: (444) 112-0106, 824-5224, ext. 217
Mobile: 044-444-447-9981
Pager: 812-7766, PIN# 9651396
Email: a_quesada_s@hotmail.com

INTERNISTS

Dr. José Luis Arenas-León
Internal Medicine, Cardiology
Address: Calle Antonio Aguilar #155,
Office V-4
Borough: Colonia Burócratas del Estado
Work: (444) 817-7013
Mobile: 044-444-803-7057
Pager: (444) 812-7766, PIN #1015291
Email: jlarenas@saludangeles.com

Dr. Jorge A. Narváes
Internal Medicine
Address: Calle Antonio Aguilar #230,
Office A-1
Borough: Colonia Burócratas del Estado
Work: (444) 811-0287
Mobile: 044-444-849-0271
Pager: 01-800-333-2223, PIN# 48490271
Email: jorgenf@lycos.com

Dr. Alejandro Quesada
Internal Medicine, Cardiopulmonary Medicine
Address: Calle Madre Perla #435,
Office 217
Borough: Fraccionamiento Indústrias
Work: (444) 112-0106, 824-5224, ext. 217
Mobile: 044-444-447-9981
Pager: 812-7766, PIN# 9651396
Email: a_quesada_s@hotmail.com

HOSPITALS

Hospital Angeles – Centro Médico del Potosí
Address: Calle Antonio Aguilar #155
Borough: Colonia Burócratas del Estado
Main Phone #: (444) 813-3797
Fax Phone #: (444) 813-1377
Emergency Phone #: (444) 813-3797,
ext. 5501
Website: www.mediks.com

Hospital Central "Dr. Ignacio Morones Prieto"
Ave. Venustiano Carranza # 2395,
Col. Universitaria
San Luis Potosí, San Luis Potosí,
Telephone (444) 834-2700 al 03

Hospital Nuestra Señora de la Salúd
Address: Calle Madre Perla #435
Borough: Fraccionamiento Indústrias
Notable Landmarks:
Close to Holiday Inn Quijote Hotel
Main Phone #: (444) 824-5224
Fax Phone #: (444) 824-5841
Emergency Phone #: (444) 824-5224,
ext. 725

SAN LUIS RIO COLORADO

GENERAL MEDICINE

Dr Felipe Martinez
Av. Padre Kino 614
Phone: (653) 4-18-14

Dr. Raul Muñoz Dominguez
5 de Mayo No. 5
Phone: (653) 4-23-43

SAN MIGUEL DE ALLENDE

CARDIOLOGISTS

Dr. Jorge Alvarez de la Cadena
Internal Medicine, Cardiology
Address: Libramiento a
Dolores Hidalgo #43, Suite 20
Borough: Colonia Mesa del Malanquín
Work: (415) 152-2320, 152-2329, 152-2233
Fax: (415) 152-5900
Mobile: 044-415-153-3131
Pager: 01-800-333-2223, PIN# 5241533131
Email: lilyjacs@unisono.net.mx

CARDIOPULMONARY MEDICINE

Dr. Roberto L. Maxwell
Internal Medicine, Emergency Medicine,
Cardiopulmonary Medicine
Address: Calle Insurgentes #29
(between Hidalgo and Reloj)
Work/Fax: (415) 152-0247
Mobile: 044-415-100-3592
Email: casamaxwell@cybermatsa.com.mx

COLPOSCOPISTS

Dra. María del Rocío Barrios
Obstetrics & Gynecology, Colposcopy
Address: Calzada de la Estación #108
Borough: Colonia Centro
Work/Fax: (415) 152-4981
Home: (415) 152-7446
Mobile: 044-415-153-5186
Email: lepanto@cybermatsa.com.mx

EAR, NOSE & THROAT

Dra. Liliana Hernández
Address: Libramiento a Dolores Hidalgo #43,
Suite 21
Borough: Colonia Mesa del Malanquín
Work: (415) 152-2329, 152-2320
Fax: (415) 152-5900
Mobile: 044-415-103-5463
Email: lilyjacs@unisono.net.mx

EMERGENCY MEDICINE

Dr. Roberto L. Maxwell
Internal Medicine, Emergency Medicine,
Cardiopulmonary Medicine
Address: Calle Insurgentes #29
(between Hidalgo and Reloj)
Work/Fax: (415) 152-0247
Mobile: 044-415-100-3592
Email: casamaxwell@cybermatsa.com.mx

GENERAL MEDICINE

Dr. Cornelio A. Hoogesteger
General Medicine, Homeopathy
Address: Callejón del Pueblito #1-A
(at corner of Reloj)
Work: (415) 152-1753

Home: (415) 152-3519
Mobile: 044-415-100-4851
Email: krelius@prodigy.net.mx

GYNECOLOGISTS

Dra. María del Rocío Barrios
Obstetrics & Gynecology, Colposcopy
Address: Calzada de la Estación #108
Borough: Colonia Centro
Work/Fax: (415) 152-4981
Home: (415) 152-7446
Mobile: 044-415-153-5186
Email: lepanto@cybermatsa.com.mx

HOMEOPATHY

Dr. Cornelio A. Hoogesteger
General Medicine, Homeopathy
Address: Callejón del Pueblito #1-A
(at corner of Reloj)
Work: (415) 152-1753
Home: (415) 152-3519
Mobile: 044-415-100-4851
Email: krelius@prodigy.net.mx

INTERNISTS

Dr. Jorge Alvarez de la Cadena
Internal Medicine, Cardiology
Address: Libramiento a Dolores Hidalgo #43,
Suite 20
Borough: Colonia Mesa del Malanquín
Work: (415) 152-2320, 152-2329, 152-2233
Fax: (415) 152-5900
Mobile: 044-415-153-3131
Pager: 01-800-333-2223, PIN# 5241533131
Email: lilyjacs@unisono.net.mx

Dr. Roberto L. Maxwell
Internal Medicine, Emergency Medicine,
Cardiopulmonary Medicine
Address: Calle Insurgentes #29
(between Hidalgo and Reloj)
Work/Fax: (415) 152-0247
Mobile: 044-415-100-3592

Email: casamaxwell@cybermatsa.com.mx

Dr. Salvador E. Quiróz
Internal Medicine, Nephrology
Address: Libramiento a Dolores Hidalgo #43,
Suite 11
Borough: Colonia Mesa del Malanquín
Work: (415) 152-2233, 152-2320, 152-2545
Fax: (415) 152-5900
Email: yolysalquiroz@prodigy.net.mx

NEPHROLOGISTS

Dr. Salvador E. Quiróz
Internal Medicine, Nephrology
Address: Libramiento a Dolores Hidalgo #43,
Suite 11
Borough: Colonia Mesa del Malanquín
Work: (415) 152-2233, 152-2320, 152-2545
Fax: (415) 152-5900
Email: yolysalquiroz@prodigy.net.mx

OBSTETRICIANS

Dra. María del Rocío Barrios
Obstetrics & Gynecology, Colposcopy
Address: Calzada de la Estación #108
Borough: Colonia Centro
Work/Fax: (415) 152-4981
Home: (415) 152-7446
Mobile: 044-415-153-5186
Email: lepanto@cybermatsa.com.mx

ORTHOPEDICIANS

Dr. Fidel G. Dobarganes
Orthopedics/Traumatology
Address: Libramiento a Dolores Hidalgo #43,
Suite 2
Borough: Colonia Mesa del Malanquín
Work: (415) 152-2233
Fax: (442) 192-3083
Mobile: (442) 281-0981
Email: fdobarganes@prodigy.net.mx
Pager: 01-800-723-4500, PIN#: 1488
Nextel: 014421253578

SURGEONS

Dr. José Diez
General Surgery
Address: Libramiento a Dolores Hidalgo #43,
Suite 3
Borough: Colonia Mesa del Malanquín
Work: (415) 152-2233, 152-2320
Fax: (415) 152-2545
Mobile: 044-415-151-7385
Nextel: 52*222*11614
Email: hospitaldelafe@prodigy.net.mx

TRAUMATOLOGISTS

Dr. Fidel G. Dobarganes
Orthopedics/Traumatology
Address: Libramiento a Dolores Hidalgo #43,
Suite 2
Borough: Colonia Mesa del Malanquín
Work: (415) 152-2233
Fax: (442) 192-3083
Mobile: (442) 281-0981
Email: fdobarganes@prodigy.net.mx
Pager: 01-800-723-4500, PIN#: 1488
Nextel: 014421253578

HOSPITALS

Hospital de la Fe
Address: Libramiento a Dolores Hidalgo, #43
Borough: Colonia Mesa del Malanquín
(a few blocks from the bus station)
Main/Fax Phone #: (415) 152-2233,
152-2320, 152-2329 (must request fax tone)
Website: www.hospitaldelafe.com

SAN NICOLAS DE LOS GARZA

HOSPITAL

Hospital Metropolitano
Dr. Bernardo Sepúlveda
Ave. López Mateos # 4600,
Col. Bosques de Nogalar
San Nicolás De Los Garza, N.L.,
Telephone (81) 8305-5900 to 39

SAN PEDRO GARZA GARCIA

AMBULANCES

EMME
Calzada San Pedro 504-A
Col. Fuentes del Valle
San Pedro Garza García, N.L.
Tel: (81) 8288-5050
Emergencies: (81) 8356-7676
Website: www.emme.com.mx

ANESTHESIOLOGISTS

Dr. Luis Fernando García Gutiérrez
Hospital CIMA Santa Engracia
Ave. Frida Kahlo 180
Col. Valle Oriente
Garza García, N.L.
Tel: (81) 8368-7777
Fax: (81) 8368-7746

DENTISTS

Dr. Roberto Carrillo
Gomez Morín 309
Col. del Valle, San Pedro Garza García
Tel: (81) 8356-5858

Dra. Alicia de León
Children's dentist
Rio Mississipi 800-A Pte.
Col. del Valle, San Pedro Garza García, N.L.
Tel: (81) 8401-5594

Dr. Albano Flores
Dental Surgery and Implants
Ricardo Margain 201
Col. Santa Engracia
San Pedro Garza García, N.L.
Tel: (81) 8378-2121

Dra. Marianela Garza
Dra. Celina Garza
Periodontics
Rio Mississipi 269-A Ote.
Col. del Valle
San Pedro Garza García, N.L.
Tel: (81) 8378-1050 / 8335-2543

Dr. Mario Garza
Adults and Children's Dentist, Orthodontics
Rio de la Plata Oriente # 101, Local H,
Col. Del Valle, San Pedro Garza García, Nuevo León, México
Office Hours M-F 10 - 19 Pm
Sat. 10 Am -13 Pm
Office (81) 8335-6562, 8400-0010
Email drmgarza@hotmail.com

Dr. Iván Garza Carrillo
Specializing In: General Dentistry & Orthodontics
Autonomous University of Nuevo León, 1962
Punto Central
Av. De la Industria # 300,
Planta Baja Local 5, Col. Veredalta
San Pedro Garza García
Office (81) 8100-9899
Home (81) 8356-0495

Dr. Juan Ángel Martinez G.
Autonomous University of Nuevo León, 1952
Mol del Valle
Calzada del Valle # 400, Despacho 818
San Pedro Garza García, Nuevo León,
Office (81) 1052-4550 / 51
Cellular 044-818-088-6962
Email perio@prodigy.net.mx

Dr. Luis Alfonso Montalvo
Specializing In: General Dentistry & Orthodontist
Autonomous University of Nuevo León, 1971
Plaza 401 Calzada Del Valle # 401,
Local E4,
Col. Del Valle, San Pedro Garza Garcia
Office (81) 1366-5757
Email ponchomotalvo@yahoo.com

Dr. Eugenio Porte
Protodontist (Prothesis)
Autonomous University of Nuevo León, 1971
Calzada San Pedro # 204 Sur,
Col. Del Valle, San Pedro Garza García,
Office (81) 8335-0215 & 8335-0132

DERMATOLOGISTS

Dr. Carlos Assad Morell
Autonomous University of Nuevo León
Clinica DermAssad, Moll Del Valle
Calzada del Valle # 400,
Planta Baja Local 44,
Col. Del Valle,
San Pedro Garza García, Nuevo León,
Office (81) 8335-7065 to 67
(81) 1768-8828
Cellular 044-811-544-4023
Email clinicadermassad@hotmail.com
Website www.dermassad.com

GYNECOLOGISTS

Dr. Pedro Tonda Ribo
Dr. Jorge A. Espinoza García
Dr. Gonzalo González Zamora
Dr. Antonio Merced Garza Garza

Dr. José Manuel Garza Leal
Dr. Leopoldo Vázquez Matute
Dr. Alejandro Calanda
Dr. Luis Gerardo Villarreal Bacco
Hospital CIMA Santa Engracia
Ave. Frida Kahlo 180
Col. Valle Oriente, Garza García, N.L.
Tel: (81) 8368-7777
Fax: (81) 8368-7746

PEDIATRICIANS

Dr. Enrique Cárdenas Ibarra
Dr. Carlos Guajardo González
Dr. Ernesto Mendoza Calderón
Hospital CIMA Santa Engracia
Ave. Frida Kahlo 180
Col. Valle Oriente
Garza García, N.L.
Tel: (81) 8368-7777
Fax: (81) 8368-7746

Dr. Gerónimo Pérez Maldonado
Hospital Santa Engracia
Av. Frida Kalo # 180, 3th Floor, Room 306,
Fracc. Valle Oriente
San Pedro Garza García, Nuevo León,
Hours: 10-12:30pm 3:30pm-7:30pm
Office (81) 8368-7805 / 06
Fax (81) 8668-7791
Email docgero@yahoo.com.mx

RADIOLOGISTS

Dr. Jorge Azpiri López
Hospital CIMA Santa Engracia
Ave. Frida Kahlo 180
Col. Valle Oriente, San Pedro Garza García,
Tel: (81) 8368-7777
Fax: (81) 8368-7746

SURGEONS

Dr. Raúl Ramos López
Dr. Alberto Chapas Lobo
Dr. Angel Martínez Vela
Dr. Francisco Treviño Garza
Hospital CIMA Santa Engracia
Ave. Frida Kahlo 180
Col. Valle Oriente, Garza García, N.L.
Tel: (81) 8368-7777
Fax: (81) 8368-7746

VETERINARIANS

Dr. Leónides Guerra Medrano
Centro Comercial Plaza Del Bosque
Av. Vasconcelos 202 #16, on the corner
of Bosques de Siberia,
San Pedro Garza García, Nuevo León,
Office (81) 8378-3414
Email drlguerra@yahoo.com

Dr. Carlos Alberto Martínez Garza
Sierra Madre Hospital Veterinario
Rio La Silla # 245, Col. Del Valle
San Pedro Garza García, Nuevo León,
Office (81) 8378-4747, 8378-4748
Email smhvet@hotmail.com

HOSPITALS

Hospital CIMA Santa Engracia
Ave. Frida Kahlo 180
Col. Valle del Mirador, San Pedro
Garza García, N.L.
Tel: (81) 8368-7777
Emergencies: (81) 8368-7731
Fax: (81) 8368-7746
Website: www.santaengracia.com

Hospital San Pedro del Valle
Av. San Pedro # 804,
Col. Fuentes Del Valle,
Telephone (81) 8378-54-00, 8378-54-66
(81) 8378-36-58, 8378-38-17
(81) 8378-36-58

SANTA ROSALIA

HOSPITAL

Clínica Hospital
Adán Velarde y Municipio Libre
(no street number)
Col. Nopalera, Santa Rosalía, B.C.S.
Tel: (615) 152-2418

TAPACHULA

HOSPITALS

Cruz Roja
9a. Norte corner with 1a. Oriente
Colonia Centro, Tapachula, Chiapas
Tel: (962) 626-1949 / 7644 / 625-3506

Hospital General
Carretera Antiguo Aeropuerto
(no street number)
Tapachula, Chiapas
Tel: (962) 628-1060 (switchboard)

TAXCO

INTERNISTS

Dr. Aaron Cohen
Address: Morelos #12
(corner of Avenida Plateros)
Borough: Colonia Centro
Work: (762) 627-3300

Home/Fax: (762) 622-8055
Mobile: 044-762-623-0083
Email: drcohenbmi@hotmail.com

PEDIATRICIAN

Dra. Luz María Trasviña
Address: Morelos #12
(corner of Avenida Plateros)
Borough: Colonia Centro
Work: (762) 622-5005, 622-3012
Fax: (762) 622-5005
Home: (762) 622-7034
Mobile: 044-762-628-0644
Email: luzmatras@hotmail.com

HOSPITALS

Clínica de Especialidades
Los Plateros 161
Col. La Misión, Taxco, Guerrero
Tel: (762) 622-4500

Clínica Santa Cruz
Address: Calle Morelos #12
Borough: Zona Centro
Notable Landmarks:
Across the street from the IMSS hospital
Main Phone #: (762) 622-3012
Fax Phone #: (762) 622-5813

Cruz Roja
Calle 2da de Jales 1
Col. Pozitos, Taxco, Guerrero
Tel: (762) 622-3232

Hospital General de Taxco "Adolfo Prieto"
Calle del Chorrillo 94
Col. Chorrillo, Taxco de Alarcón, Guerrero
Tel: (762) 622-9300

TEPATITLAN

HOSPITAL

Sanatorio Medico Quirurgico de los Altos
Bartolo Hernandez 250
Tel. 01 (378) 782-1243
Emergencies: 24 hours

TEPIC

HOSPITALS - PRIVATE

Centro Quirurgico San Rafael
(medical specialties,surgery emergency
care, ICU)
Avenida del Valle 91
Colonia Ciudad del Valle, Tepic, Nayarit
Tel: (311) 214-1146

Clinica Dental Nayar
Mexico 161 Norte
Col. Centro, Tepic, Nayarit
Tel: (311) 212-2827

Consultorio Cardiologico Nayarit
Avenida Juan Escutia 82 Norte
Tepic, Nayarit
Tel. & Fax: (311) 212-3152

Sanatorio La Loma
H. Colegio Militar 361 Sur
Colonia Centro, Tepic, Nayarit
Tel. 01 (311) 213-2013
Emergencies: 24 hours

Unidad Medica Tepic Nayarit (by appointment)
(311) 214-6898
(311) 214-9255 & (311) 213-4568

HOSPITALS - PUBLIC

Cruz Roja Mexicana
Insurgentes y Rey Nayar
Col. 12 de diciembre, Tepic, Nayarit
Tel: (311) 214-6635
Emergencies: (311) 213-1160

Hospital General de TEPIC
Ave. Enfermeria (no street number)
Col. Centro, Tepic, Nayarit
Tel: (311) 213-7937 / 4127
Emergencies: (311) 214-2315 / 3291

Sanatorío Guadalupe
Juan Escutia 68 Norte
Tepic, Nayarit
Tel. & Fax: (311) 212-9401 / 2713

TIJUANA

EMERGENCY NUMBERS

Excel Hospital,
Avenida Paseo de Los Héroes # 2507,
Zona del Rio, Tijuana, B.C
México tel: 664-634-3434
Hospital del Prado,
Calle Bugambilias # 50,
Fraccionamiento El Prado,
Tijuana, B.C. CP 22105
Mexico tel: 664-681-4900

Hospital del Carmen,
Calle Manuel Doblado #402,
Colonia Gabilondo, Tijuana, B.C.
México tel: 664-681-7279

Scripps Mercy Hospital,
435 H Street, Chula Vista,
California, 91910, United States,
Tel: (619) 691-7000

GENERAL MEDICINE

Dr. Guillermo Uribe
Centro Médico del Noroeste
Blvd. Sánchez Taboada
Esq. Misión de San Diego # 1527-205
Zona del Río
684-8127, 634-7788
e-mail: drguribe@hotmail.com

ALLERGISTS

Dr. Alfredo Ramírez Olivo
Blvd. Agua Caliente #1844-203
684-7918

CARDIOLOGISTS

Dr. Patricia Aubanel
Calle Bugambilias #50, Oficina 202
Fraccionamiento el Prado
Tel: (664) 621-0262, 681-4900
Fax: (664) 621-0263, 621-0262
Cel: (664) 161-8582
e-mail: icchp@telnor.net

Dr. Arturo Guerra
Centro Médico Lucerna
Germán Gedovious 10431 - 202
Zona Río, Tijuana, Baja California
Tel. & Fax: (664) 684-2989/0169
Cell: (664) 628-7447

Dr. Juan José Parcero
German Gedovious No. 9506-302
Zona Río, Tijuana, Baja California
Tel. & Fax: (664) 684-7568, 634-7482
Avenida Paseo de los Héroes #10999,
Office 511, Zona Rio
Tel: (664) 634-7482, 634-7568
Fax: (664) 634-2560
Cel: 044-664-628-5442
e-mail: jjpv59@prodigy.net.mx

Dr. Jaime Sánchez Salazar
Misión Santo Tomas #1515
Zona del Río
684-2934

DENTISTS

Dr. Ricardo Alvarez O.
Misión de Loreto #3045
Zona Río
smile@dental.alvarez.com

Dr. Sergio Araiza
Misión de Mulegé No. 2910
Zona Río, Tijuana, Baja California
Tel. & Fax: (664) 634-3410

Dr. Rogelio Hernández
Misión de San Diego 1527-102
Zona Río, Tijuana, Baja California
Tel. & Fax: (664) 634-3639 / 3699

Dr. Javier Valdez Aceves
Calle 7ma. Galeana # 7971
Zona Centro
drjaviervaldez@yahoo.com.mx
681-3516
U.S.: (619) 734-0222
688-1575
685-3123

DERMATOLOGISTS

Dr. Raul Ahumada
Blvd. Agua Caliente # 4558, Suite 1303
Centro Dermatológico de Tijuana
Doctor.ahumada3@gmail.com
686-5406
686-5420
U.S: 619-754-4971

EAR, NOSE & THROAT

Dr. Hector Delgadillo
Bugambilias No. 50-403
Hospital del Prado

Dr. Humberto Luna Gonzalez
José Clemente Orozco #10122
Suite 204
Playa Pacifico
681-4900 x2403
Fax: 681-1984
684-9333
684-8844

ENDOCRINOLOGISTS

Dr. Juan Ceballos Hernandez
Gobernador Lugo # 9815
Consultorio No. 207
Col. Gabilondo
686-3126
686-4238
Fax: 686-5681
Jceballos76@hotmail.com

GYNECOLGISTS

Dra. Estela Behr y Rico
Av. Centenario de Tijuana # 10310-206
Edificio Cazar
Zona del Río
e-mail: ursulabehr@yahoo.com

Dr. Francisco Díaz Martínez
Calle Cuarta #8193
Entre Revolución y Constitución
Zona Centro

Dra. Martha Gassol
Jose Ma. Velazco #2613-103
Edif. Centro Profesional del Río
Entre Paseo de los Héroes y Sánchez
Taboada, Zona del Río
Tel: 664-634-3879

Dr. Alejandro Padilla Fitch
Centro Médico Tijuana
Gobernador Lugo 3003-301
Colonia Gabilondo
Urgency Hospital del Carmen
Tijuana, Baja California
Tel. & Fax:(664) 686-1648

Dr. Arturo H. Rosas Prianti
Bugambilias #50-205 2do piso
Fraccionamiento El Prado
Tel: (664) 681-6382
Home: (664) 630-1155
Cel: (664) 628-5747

INTERNISTS

Dr. Jorge Astiazaran Orci
Torres Agua Caliente
Blvd. Agua Caliente No. 4558-9, Nivel C
Tijuana, Baja California
Tel. & Fax: (664) 686-1030,
683-3000 code 660413

Dr. Patricia Aubanel
Calle Bugambilias #50, Oficina 202
Fraccionamiento el Prado
Tel: (664) 621-0262, 681-4900
Fax: (664) 621-0263, 621-0262
Cel: (664) 161-8582
e-mail: icchp@telnor.net

Dr. Rodolfo Chávez Pardo
Hospital Angeles
Ave. Sánchez Taboada 10999-505
Zona Río, Tijuana, Baja California
Tel. & Fax: (664) 635-1888 / 1900

Dr. Héctor Zepeda
Avenida Paseo de los Héroes #10999,
Oficina 809
Col. Zona Río
Tel: (664) 635-1847
Cel: (664) 628-4142
e-mail: hectorzepeda@gmail.com

NEUROLOGISTS

Dr. Hugo Navarrete Báez
Abelardo L. Rodríguez #2916
Altos A-2, Zona del Río
684-0687
e-mail: doctorhugo@gmail.com

NEUROSUGERONS

Dr. Jose Luis Pizano
Central Médica de Especialistas
Blvd. Agua Caliente #1844
Consultorio 304
664-684-7824
e-mail: pizanol@yahoo.com

Dr. Carlos Ruíz Macías
Paseo de los Héroes #10999
Consultorio 205, 2do piso
Zona Rio
Hospital Angeles Tijuana
684-7824
Cell: 620-7777
635-1809
Cell: 648-9364
e-mail: Neuro667@hotmail.com

OBSTETRICS

Dr. Arturo H. Rosas
Calle Bugambilias #50, Office 205
Fraccionamiento El Prado
Tel: (664) 681-6382
Home: (664) 630-1155
Cel: (664) 628-5747

OPHTALMOLOGISTS

Dr. Jorge Angel Bórquez P.
Bugambilias #50-501
Hospital del Prado
Cell: 681-6014
681-4900 x2501

ORTHOPEDICS

Dr. Dario Garin
Avenida Paseo de los Héroes #109,
Office 301, Zona Rio
Tel: (664) 635-1813 or 635-1800,
ext. 4301, 4302
Cel: 044-664-693-3665
e-mail: dgarinmd@hotmail.com

PEDIATRICIANS

Dr. Pedro Gabriel Chong King
Avenida Paseo de los Héroes #10999,
Office 101
Zona Río
Tel/Fax: (664) 608-9096 or 635-1801,
ext. 4101
Cel: (664) 666-1483
e-mail: pgchk@yahoo.com

Dr. José Luis Gaitán Morán
Unidad de Pediatría Médica
Erasmo Castellano y
Blvd. Sánchez Taboada #18
Suite 114, Zona Rio
e-mail: pepegaitan@hotmail.com

Dr. Eduardo Sáenz Urquidi
Centro Médico del Noroeste
Blvd. Sánchez Taboada y
Misión de San Diego No.
2993 Int. 107
Zona del Río
635-1801
Cell: 666-1483
684-7915
Fax: 634-0886
634-1810
Cell: 693-2838
e-mail: saenzedr@hotmail.com

Dr. Jorge T. Tsutsumi
Calle Bugambilias #50, Office 305
Fraccionamiento El Prado
Tel: (664) 681-6556
Home: (664) 686-5709
Cel: (664) 639-0469
e-mail: jttsutsumi@yahoo.com

PLASTIC SURGEONS

Dr. Jaime Caloca
Abelardo L. Rodríguez #10-201
Zona del Río
Tel: 734-2246
e-mail: drcaloca@drcaloca.com

Dr. Benito Rodríguez López
Clínica de Cirugía Plástica
Diego Rivera #2550
Zona del Río
634-2090
634-2359
634-2307
634-2308
686-4356
e-mail: drbenitorodriguez1@hotmail.com

RADIOLOGISTS

Dr. Jaime A. Saldaña
German Gedovious #7
Centro Médico Lucerna
Zona del Río
684-0948
684-1908
rxlucerna@hotmail.com

SURGEON (GENERAL, TRAUMA)

Dr. Sergio P. Mascareño
Avenida Paseo de los Héroes #10999,
Office 607
Zona Rio
Tel: (664) 635-1834 or 635-1800, ext. 4607
Home: (664) 621-8376
Cel: 044-664-628-7466
e-mail: serquir@yahoo.com

UROLOGISTS

Dr. Daniel Armendáriz Beltrán
Brasilia #12928
Fracc. El Paraíso
621-0658
Fax: 621-0673
e-mail: Dr_armendariz@msn.com

HOSPITALS

Hospital Angeles
Avenida Paseo de los Héroes #10999
Colonia Zona Río
Tel: (664) 635-1900
Fax: (664) 635-1917
e-mail: czavala@saludangeles.com
Website: www.medlinks.com

Hospital del Carmen
Manuel Doblado 402
Colonia Gabilondo, Tijuana, Baja California
Tel: (664) 681-7279 (6 lines)
Fax: (664) 686-2525

Hospital deL Prado
Bugambilias No. 50
Fracc. Prado, Tijuana, Baja California
Tel: (664) 681-4900 to 03
Fax: (664) 681-6540
Emergency phone: (664) 621-0919
English help line: (664) 621-0917
e-mail: hospitaldelprado@hotmail.com

Hospital Excell
(Specialized, with Critical and Intensive Care
Units for open heart surgery)
Paseo de los Héroes No. 2507
Zona Río, Tijuana, Baja California
Tel. & Fax: (664) 634-7002/7001/3434

TORREON

HOSPITAL

Hospital Universitario
Ave. Juárez #951 Oriente,
Zona Centro Torreón,
Coahuila de Zaragoza,
Telephone (871) 713-4416 & 713-4833
Fax (871) 722-0897

TUXTLA GUTIERREZ

GENERAL PRACTITIONERS

Dr. Carlso Camacho Escobar
15 Poniente Norte 167
Col. Moctezuma, Tuxtla Gutiérrez, Chiapas
Tel: (961) 602-5807

Dra. Ana Marcela Pizañas
Unidad Médica Metropolitana
7a Norte Oriente 175
Tuxtla Gutiérrez, Chiapas
Tel: (961) 614-8097

Dr. Juan Alberto Zarza Castro
5 Poniente Sur 159, Office 101
Colonia Centro, Tuxtla Gutiérrez, Chiapas
Tel: (961) 613-6652

DENTISTS

Dr. Edmundo Diaz Ordaz
Dra. Patricia Diaz Ordaz
15 Poniente Norte 245
Colonia Moctezuma
Tuxtla Gutierrez, Chiapas
Tel: (961) 602-5793 / 5796
Cell (961) 602-0770

GYNECOLOGISTS

Dr. Valdemar A. Rojas
Obstetrics & Gynecology
Address: Calle "14 Poniente" Sur #365,
4th floor
Borough: Colonia Centro
Work/Fax: (961) 121-4913
Home: (961) 612-0232
Mobile: 044-961-102-0107

INTERNISTS

Dr. Leopoldo Niño
Internal Medicine
Address: Calle "14a Poniente" Sur #365,
1st floor
Work/Fax: (961) 602-9675
Mobile: 044-961-655-4111
Email: leopoldonino@infosel.net.mx

OBSTETRICIANS

Dr. Valdemar A. Rojas
Obstetrics & Gynecology
Address: Calle "14 Poniente" Sur #365,
4th floor
Borough: Colonia Centro
Work/Fax: (961) 121-4913
Home: (961) 612-0232
Mobile: 044-961-102-0107

PEDIATRICIAN

Dr. German R. Muench
Pediatrics & Pediatric Surgery
Address: Calle "15 Poniente" Norte, #190 Altos
Borough: Colonia Moctezuma
Work/Fax: (961) 602-5997
Mobile: 044-961-649-0628
Email: gemuna@prodigy.net.mx

SURGEONS

Dr. Marco A. Castillo
General Surgery
Address: Calle "Primera Sur" Poniente #232,
1st floor
Borough: Colonia Centro
Work: (961) 612-0911
Home: (961) 613-1484
Mobile: 044-961-579-2226
Email: castillo_marcoanto@hotmail.com, castillo_marcoanto@terra.com.mx

HOSPITALS

Centro Medico Ana Isabel (Private)
1 Sur Poniente 725
Colonia Centro, Tuxtla Gutiérrez, Chiapas
Tel: (961) 612-2334 / 2293

Cruz Roja -Municipal
15a. Ave. Norte Poniente 1480
Between 14 and 13 Poniente
Zona Centro, Tuxtla Gutiérrez, Chiapas
Tel: (961) 612-9514 / 0492

Hospital General
Regional "Dr. Rafael Pascacio Gamboa"
9a. Sur Oriente (no street number)
Colonia Centro, Tuxtla Gutiérrez, Chiapas
Tel: (961) 613-0047 / 0099

Sanatorío Rojas (Private)
2 Sur Poniente 1487
Colonia La Lomita, Tuxtla Gutiérrez, Chiapas
Tel & Fax: (961) 602-5138 / 5024

Sanatorio Rojas
Address: Calle "2a. Sur" Poniente #1487
Borough: Colonia La Lomita
Main/Fax Phone #: (961) 602-5004, 602-5024
Emergency Phone #: (961) 602-5138,
602-5128

URUAPAN

HOSPITALS

Cruz Roja
Lago y Jacarandas 1
Fracc. Hurtado, Uruapan, Michoacán
Tel: (452) 524-1588

Hospital General Regional de Uruapan "Dr. Pedro Daniel Martinez"
Camino a Tejerías Km. 1.5
Col. San Francisco, Uruapan, Michoacán
Tel: (452) 528-0256

VERACRUZ

GYNECOLOGISTS

Dra. Silvia Váldes
Obstetrics & Gynecology
Address: Avenida Cuahutémoc #2358
(corner of Calle Cuba)
Office: (229) 934-2618
Mobile: 044-229-126-3199

INTERNISTS

Dr. Raymundo Orla
Address: Calle "16 de Septiembre" #955
Borough: Colonia Centro
Work: (229) 931-3902
Fax: (229) 932-9183
Mobile: 044-229-929-2288
Email: ray@sbd.ver.megared.net.mx

OBSTETRICIANS

Dra. Silvia Váldes
Obstetrics & Gynecology
Address: Avenida Cuahutémoc #2358
(corner of Calle Cuba)
Office: (229) 934-2618
Mobile: 044-229-126-3199

PEDIATRICIANS

Dr. Rafael B. Díaz
Pediatrics, Neonatology
Address: Calle "16 de Septiembre" #955,
Office 2

Borough: Colonia Centro
Work: (229) 931-3902
Mobile: 044-229-928-7108
Email: dr_diazsalcedo@hotmail.com

HOSPITALS

Hospital de la Sociedad Española de
Beneficencia de Veracruz (Hospital Español)
Address: Calle "16 de Septiembre" #955
(between Escobedo and Abasolo streets)
Borough: Colonia Centero
Notable Landmarks: Six blocks from city center
Main Phone #: (229) 932-1282
Fax Phone #: (229) 932-1100
Emergency Phone #: (229) 931-4000

VILLAHERMOSA

ENDOCRINOLOGISTS

Dr. Mauro V. Carrillo
Internal Medicine, Endocrinology
Address: Prolongación Avenida Paseo
Usumacinta #2085, Office 402
Borough: Colonia Tabasco 2000
Work: (993) 316-1231
Fax: (993) 316-6999
Mobile: 044-993-160-5923
Email: mvcarvel1@yahoo.com.mx

GYNECOLOGISTS

Dr. Manuel González
Obstetrics & Gynecology
Address: Prolongación Avenida Paseo
Usumacinta #2085, Office 453
Borough: Colonia Tabasco 2000
Work/Fax: (993) 316-9535
Mobile: 044-993-311-3631
Email: manglez@prodigy.net.mx

INTERNISTS

Dr. Mauro V. Carrillo
Internal Medicine, Endocrinology
Address: Prolongación Avenida Paseo
Usumacinta #2085, Office 402
Borough: Colonia Tabasco 2000
Work: (993) 316-1231
Fax: (993) 316-6999
Mobile: 044-993-160-5923
Email: mvcarvel1@yahoo.com.mx

NEONATOLOGISTS

Dr. Humberto Martínez-García
Pediatrics, Neonatology
Address: Prolongación Avenida Paseo
Usumacinta #2085, Office 334A
Borough: Colonia Tabasco 2000
Work: (993) 316-0207
Fax: (993) 316-6999
Home: (993) 316-4107
Mobile: 044-993-391-1495
Email: beto_m_g@msn.com

OBSTETRICIANS

Dr. Manuel González
Obstetrics & Gynecology
Address: Prolongación Avenida Paseo
Usumacinta #2085, Office 453
Borough: Colonia Tabasco 2000
Work/Fax: (993) 316-9535
Mobile: 044-993-311-3631
Email: manglez@prodigy.net.mx

ORTHOPEDICS

Dr. Pedro B. Cáceres
Orthopedics/Traumatology
Address: Prolongación Avenida
Paseo Usumacinta #2085, Office 350
Borough: Colonia Tabasco 2000
Work/Fax: (993) 316-7000
Mobile: 044-993-311-5243
Email: pcaceres@saludangeles.com

PEDIATRICIANS

Dr. Humberto Martínez-García
Pediatrics, Neonatology
Address: Prolongación Avenida Paseo
Usumacinta #2085, Office 334A
Borough: Colonia Tabasco 2000
Work: (993) 316-0207
Fax: (993) 316-6999
Home: (993) 316-4107
Mobile: 044-993-391-1495
Email: beto_m_g@msn.com

TRAUMATOLOGISTS

Dr. Pedro B. Cáceres
Orthopedics/Traumatology
Address: Prolongación Avenida Paseo
Usumacinta #2085, Office 350
Borough: Colonia Tabasco 2000
Work/Fax: (993) 316-7000
Mobile: 044-993-311-5243
Email: pcaceres@saludangeles.com

HOSPITALS

Hospital Angeles-Villahermosa
Address: Prolongación Avenida Paseo
Usumacinta #2085
Borough: Colonia Tabasco 2000
Notable Landmarks: Next to Pemex Gas
and Petroquimica Básica
Main Phone #: (993) 316-7000
Fax Phone #: (993) 316-6999
Emergency #: (993) 316-7000, ext. 1

ZACATECAS

HOSPITAL

Centro Hospitalario de San José
Plaza Constitución # 208,
Col. Centro, Zacatecas,
Zacatecas, México
Teléfono (492) 922-0226
Fax (492) 922-0226 ext. 200

ZAMORA

NEUROLOGIST/ NEUROSURGEON

Dr. Alejandro Méndez Dávalos
Virrey de Almanza 4 Int. 201
Fracc. La Luneta
Zamora, Michoacán
Tel: (351) 512-1060
Fax: (351) 512-2345

HOSPITALS

Cruz Roja
Virrey de Mendoza 447
Col. Jardinadas
Zamora, Michoacán
Tel: (351) 512-0534 / 0535

Hospital General de Zamora
Prol. 5 de Mayo Norte 97
Fracc. Jardines de Jericó
Zamora, Michoacán
Tel: (351) 517-7482

ZAPOPAN

DENTISTS

Dr. Hector Haro D.D.S.
Empresarios 3514 150-1105
Zapopan, Jalisco
Tel: 3848-5551 / 3848-5561 / 3813-0129

Dr. Veronica Valdez Lopez
Tchaikovsky 253-A
Col. La Estancia, Zapopan, Jal.
Tels: 3629-7860, 1204-4898 & 1204-4899
Cel: 044-333-198-2788

Dr. Abraham Waxstein Nudelstejer
Office: Av. Mexico 2309-1
Zapopan, Jalisco
Tel: 3615-1041 / 3615-3260

GASTROENTEROLOGISTS

Dr. Fernando Aceves Miramontes
Blvd. Puerto de Hierro #5150
Centro Médico Puerta de Hierro
Torre "C", Piso 2 Consultorio 201-C
Zapopan, Jal.
Tel: 3813-1685 3813-1696
Cel: 044-333-189-0744

PEDIATRICIANS

Dr. Jaime Julio Unda Gomez
Office: Av. Empresarios 150 - 8th floor
Zapopan, Jalisco
Tel: 3848-5520
Cel: 044-333-157-8511

PLASTIC SURGEONS

Dr. Rene C. Mora Esquivias
Office: Lapizlazuli 3050
Zapopan, Jalisco
Tel: 3647-42-69 / 3628-70-79
Celular: 0443-662-5042

UROLOGISTS

Dr. Jaime Vargas Basterra
Office: Blvd. Puerta de Hierro No. 5150
Torre B
Zapopan, Jalisco
Tel: 3848-5497 / 3848-5498 / 3848-4000
Cel: 044-333-137-9247

HOSPITALS

Centro Médico Puerta de Hierro
Plaza Corporativa Zapopan
Empresarios 150
Zapopan, Jalisco
Tel: (33) 3848-2100
Website: http://www.cmpdh.com/

Hospital "Angel Leaño"
Av. Dr. Angel Leaño 500
Zapopan, Jalisco
Tel: 3648-8425 / 3648-8484

Hospital Puerta de Hierro
Av. Empresarios # 150
Zapopan Jalisco
Tel. 01800 263 CMPDH
Tel. 01(33) 3848 4000
http://www.cmpdh.com/

Hospital Real San Jose

Ave. Lázaro Cárdenas No. 4149
Jardines de San Ignacio
Zapopan, Jalisco
Tel. 1078-8900
http://www.hrsj.com.mx/en/

Hospital Santa Maria Chapalita
Av. Niño Obrero 1666
Col. Chapalita, Zapopan, Jalisco
Tel: 3678-1400
hsmchap@prodigy.net.mx

ZIHUATANEJO

CARDIOLOGISTS

Dr. Armando Rosas-Pineda
Internal Medicine, Cardiology
Address: Calle Las Palmas #40
Borough: Colonia Centro
Town: Zihuatanejo
Work/Fax: (755) 554-0517
Mobile: 044-755-100-6005
Email: armandorosaspineda@hotmail.com

INTERNISTS

Dr. Natalio Molina
Internal Medicine
Address: Avenida La Parota #8
(at the corner of Calle Los Hujes)
Borough: Colonia El Hujal
Town: Zihuatanejo
Work: (755) 554-6838, 554-7628
Home: (755) 554-0524
Mobile: 044-755-557-0918

Dr. Armando Rosas-Pineda
Internal Medicine, Cardiology
Address: Calle Las Palmas #40
Borough: Colonia Centro
Town: Zihuatanejo

Work/Fax: (755) 554-0517
Mobile: 044-755-100-6005
Email: armandorosaspineda@hotmail.com

GYNECOLOGISTS

Dr. Juan Jose Tellez Castro
Obstetrics & Gynecology
Address: Avenida La Parota #8
(At the corner of Calle Los Hujes)
Borough: Colonia El Hujal, Zihuatanejo
Work/Fax: (755) 554-3947
Home: (755) 554-2424
Mobile: 044-755-558-8413
Email: teca15@hotmail.com

OBSTETRICIANS

Dr. Juan J. Téllez
Obstetrics & Gynecology
Address: Avenida La Parota #8
(At the corner of Calle Los Hujes)
Borough: Colonia El Hujal, Zihuatanejo
Work/Fax: (755) 554-3947
Home: (755) 554-2424
Mobile: 044-755-558-8413
Email: teca15@hotmail.com

OPHTHALMOLOGISTS

Dr. Miguel Angel Diego Berdeja
Calle Nicolás Bravo 210-27
Col. Centro, Zihuatanejo, Guerrero
Tel: (755) 554-0701

PEDIATRICIAN

Dr. Valente Real
Pediatrics, Pediatric Surgery
Address: Andador #38, Lote 5, Mza 12
Borough: Fraccionamiento Mira Flores
Town: Zihuatanejo
Work: (755) 554-2882
Fax: (755) 755-554-5112
Mobile: 044-755-557-0329
Email: drreal@prodigy.net.mx

HOSPITALS

Clínica Maciel
Calle de la Palma 12
Col. Centro, Zihuatanejo, Guerrero
Tel & Fax: (755) 554-2380 / 0517

Cruz Roja
Ave. de las Huertas 116
Col. Centro, Zihuatanejo, Guerrero
Tel: (755) 554-2009
Administration: (755) 554-9432 / 6533

Hospital de Especialidades Zihuatanejo
Address: Avenida la Parota
(at the corner of Calle Los Hujes)
Notable Landmarks: Near the bus station and
Fuente del Sol Monument
Borough: Colonia El Hujal
Zihuatanejo, Guerrero
Main Phone #: (755) 554-7628, 554-6808
Fax Phone #: (755) 554-6961

Hospital Dr. Hernandez Montejano
24 Hour Emergency Services
Juan N. Alvarez (no street number)
corner with Benito Juárez
Col. Centro, Zihuatanejo, Guerrero
Tel: (755) 554-5404
Fax: (755) 554-8703

Hospital General Regional
"Dr. Bernardo Sepúlveda Gutiérrez"
Paseo Zihuatanejo
corner with Mar Egeo
Zihuatanejo, Guerrero
Tel: (755) 554-3436
Fax: (755) 554-3650

ZINAPECUARO

HOSPITAL

Centro de Salud
Hidalgo (no street number)
Zinapécuaro, Michoacán
Tel. (451) 355-0015

ABOUT THE AUTHORS

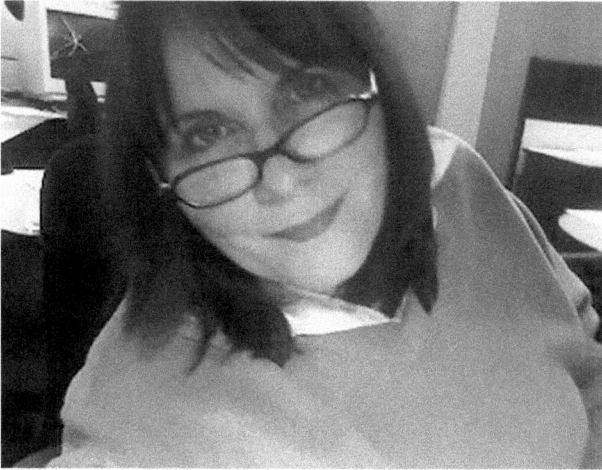

Monica Rix Paxson *is an award-winning author writing on topics related to science and medicine including the book* The English Speaker's Guide to Medical Care in Mexico. *She has appeared on CNN, Good Morning America, CBS This Morning and the BBC.*

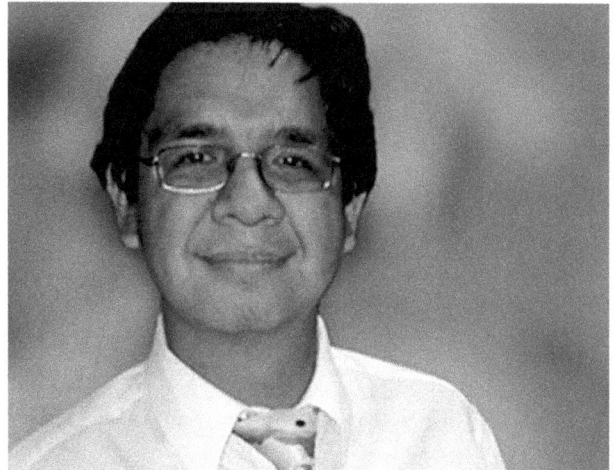

Luis Felipe Garcia Perez *has a Master's Degree in International Commerce. He is fluent in English, Spanish, and French and has lived in Mexico, Canada, and France. He's a freelancer writer and has researched and written extensively about medicine and the health care system in Mexico.*

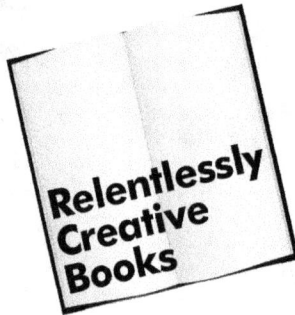

Relentlessly Creative Books™ offers an exciting new publishing option for authors. Our "middle path publishing™" approach includes many of the advantages of both traditional publishing and self-publishing without the drawbacks. For more information and a complete online catalog of our books, please visit us at RelentlesslyCreative.com. or write us at books@relentlesslycreative.com.

For readers, join our online **Readers Group** and enjoy free eBooks, sneak previews on new releases, book sales, author interviews, book reviews, reader surveys and online events with Authors. Register at RelentlesslyCreative.com.

www.ingramcontent.com/pod-product-compliance
Lightning Source LLC
Chambersburg PA
CBHW081416270326
41931CB00015B/3299